P9-CJQ-717

A Personal Chef Cooks:

Recipes from a Decade of Lower Fat Cooking

By

Cheryl Y. Mochau

Library Resource Center
Renton Technical College
3000 N.E. 4th St.
Renton, WA 98056

© 2003 by Cheryl Y. Mochau. All rights reserved.

No part of this book may be reproduced, stored in a retrieval system, or transmitted by any means, electronic, mechanical, photocopying, recording, or otherwise, without written permission from the author.

ISBN: 1-4033-2952-4 (e-book)
ISBN: 1-40332-953-2 (Paperback)

This book is printed on acid free paper.

641.5638 MOCHAU 2003

Mochau, Cheryl.

A personal chef cooks

1stBooks - rev. 12/18/02

Dedication

This book is dedicated to God, who blesses us daily in so many ways.

About The Book

This cookbook has come about from more than a decade of cooking fat reduced meals for my clients. As a personal chef, I have had the pleasure of preparing health-restoring foods for people with a variety of dietary concerns, especially helping clients achieve a lower fat lifestyle by reducing their daily fat intake. Along the way, the most common request by far was to re-create favorite comfort foods that were lower in fat than the originals — but still tasty!

Whether your tastes range from chicken to chocolate, there are slimmed down new favorites waiting for you in this collection of one hundred recipes. Fill pita pockets with the South of the Border Salmon Filling or surprise a wheat-intolerant friend with Wheat Free Coffee Cake. Enjoy your old favorite, Chicken Divan, slimmed down in fat, but not in taste, and remember to share the Lemon Tarts that will have you wondering why we ever put butter in them in the first place. This collection is just what you need for fun favorites without all the fat.

Many of the ideas for these recipes have come from my clients' favorite family memories, cookbooks, and magazines, or from memorable restaurant dishes that have been described in great detail. As I captured and tested each recipe, I reflected on the many people who have enjoyed them in the past. Few things delight me more than remembering their smiling faces recounting enjoyable dinner scenes.

My husband, Geoff, has faithfully tasted every single dish and has been instrumental in helping this collection take shape. I am grateful to him and to all who have helped to make this book possible.

Cheryl Y. Mochau
December 9, 2002

Table of Contents

Recipes

I do not consider myself a particularly creative cook. However, occasionally the time and place and direction of the sun are just right and new ideas are born.

There have been times when I've headed for the kitchen with crazy ideas of making some fabulous dish only to be limited by whatever is in the cupboard and winding up with an entirely different taste and look. When this happens I simultaneously write two recipes: the current one under construction and the one that originally provoked it. Later, when I can get the right ingredients from the market, the second one becomes a reality.

This is sometimes a thing of beauty and other times simply worthy of the disposal. It is, however, one of the many ways that I have learned to express a joyful life.

<u>Recipe Notes</u>

- Preparation times are in the form: Hours: Minutes.
- Ingredients are typically listed in the order they are used and may appear multiple times if used in separate steps.
- Water is sometimes (but not always) listed as an ingredient.
- All nutritional information is calculated per serving.
- "CFF" is "Calories From Fat".

Disclaimer
This cookbook is not intended as a specific diet or weight loss plan. Always consult a physician and registered dietitian with specific dietary concerns. The nutritional information provided is believed to be accurate, but is not guaranteed.

STARTERS

Cheryl Mochau

Bean 'n' Cheese Bites

Serves: 12   Preparation Time: 0:45

Amount	Measure	Ingredient — Preparation Method
¾	cup	fat free refried beans
2	tablespoons	onions — finely chopped
2	tablespoons	salsa
2	cups	reduced fat buttermilk baking mix
1	cup	light sour cream
1	teaspoon	onion powder
2	tablespoons	chili peppers — minced
2	tablespoons	sweet red pepper — minced
¾	cup	reduced fat Monterey jack cheese — shredded
½	teaspoon	chili powder

Preheat oven to 375°.

Mix the refried beans, onions and salsa together, reserve. In a separate bowl combine the baking mix, sour cream and onion powder. Knead for 1 minute then roll out ¼" thick, adding more baking mix as needed to prevent sticking. Cut in 2" circles, place on an ungreased cookie sheet and press an indent in the center of each circle with your thumb. Smooth a teaspoon of the bean paste in the center, leaving the edges of the crust exposed. Top with the green chilies, red peppers, cheese and a dusting of chili powder.

Bake for 12-15 minutes or until golden brown. Makes 24.

NOTES: These freeze well in covered plastic ware when stacked between sheets of waxed paper. To serve, just thaw and reheat in a 400° oven for 5 minutes.

This recipe originated from Betty Crocker's Creative Bisquick® Recipes and has been lightened up with low fat products.

110 Calories; 3g Fat (22% CFF); 5g Protein; 17g Carbohydrate; 4mg Cholesterol; 364mg Sodium

Candied Kielbasa

Serves: 16   Preparation Time: 0:20

Amount	Measure	Ingredient — Preparation Method
1	tablespoon	margarine
1	pound	turkey kielbasa
½	cup	brown sugar
1	teaspoon	onion powder

Melt the margarine in a large skillet over medium-high heat.

Cut the kielbasa into ¼" pennies and cook for 4-5 minutes (until browned). Reduce the temperature to medium, add the brown sugar and onion powder, stirring constantly until the sugar dissolves. Reduce the temperature to low, simmer, stirring frequently for 8-10 minutes. Serve hot.

NOTES: A version of this recipe appeared in a 1999 Gluten Free newsletter. If using non-turkey kielbasa, drain off all but 1 tablespoon of fat and omit the margarine before adding the sugar and flavoring.

93 Calories; 5g Fat (50% CFF); 4g Protein; 8g Carbohydrate; 20mg Cholesterol; 296mg Sodium

Shrimp Toasts

Serves: 15   Preparation Time: 0:50

Amount	Measure	Ingredient — Preparation Method
30	slices	party-style white bread
6	ounces	cooked shrimp — peeled, cleaned
$\frac{1}{4}$	teaspoon	lemon juice
1	tablespoon	onions — minced fine
4	ounces	Swiss cheese — minced
$\frac{1}{8}$	teaspoon	black pepper
1 $\frac{1}{2}$	tablespoons	mayonnaise
$\frac{1}{8}$	teaspoon	paprika

Preheat oven to broil.

Using a sharp knife, trim the crusts away from the loaf of bread, leaving 1 ½" rounds. Place on a broiler pan and lightly toast one side under the broiler. Remove from the oven and turn the toasts over, set aside.

Reduce the oven temperature to 375°.

Chop the shrimp fine, combine with the remaining ingredients — except the paprika. Place 1 teaspoon of the filling on each toast round. Sprinkle with paprika.

Bake for 3-4 minutes or until the cheese melts. Makes 30.

NOTES: These freeze well just prior to baking. Put the baking sheet filled with a single layer of unbaked Shrimp Toasts in the freezer for 30 minutes. Remove and layer them between sheets of waxed paper and store in plastic ware. To serve, thaw in a single layer on a baking sheet for 30 minutes, bake in a preheated 375° oven for 3-4 minutes or until the cheese melts and the edges are crispy.

This recipe came my way from a client who loves to entertain. She always keeps several packages of these in the freezer ready for guests.

184 Calories; 5g Fat (26% CFF); 8g Protein; 25g Carbohydrate; 30mg Cholesterol; 321mg Sodium

Picadillo Dip

	Serves: 8	Preparation Time: 0:30

Amount	Measure	Ingredient — Preparation Method
$\frac{1}{2}$	cup	onions — minced
$\frac{1}{4}$	cup	green pepper — minced
$\frac{1}{4}$	cup	sweet red pepper — minced
1	tablespoon	garlic — minced
1	pound	ground chicken breast
14	ounces	tomatoes, canned — with juice
$\frac{1}{4}$	cup	raisins — chopped
$\frac{2}{3}$	cup	dill pickles — chopped, with juice
1	tablespoon	green olives — sliced
2	tablespoons	brown sugar
1	teaspoon	chili powder
1	teaspoon	grainy Dijon mustard
$\frac{1}{4}$	teaspoon	pumpkin pie spice
$\frac{1}{8}$	teaspoon	black pepper

Lightly coat a skillet with vegetable cooking spray and place over medium-high heat. Sauté the onion and peppers for 3 minutes. Add the garlic and ground chicken. Sauté about 5 minutes, breaking the chicken into small bits with a spatula. Stir in the remaining ingredients. Reduce the heat to simmer for 15 minutes or until the liquid is almost all evaporated, but still moist.

Serve hot with snack crackers or fresh vegetable wedges.

NOTES: Get more flavor out of the raisins by chopping them coarsely.
Pumpkin pie spice is a combination of cinnamon, nutmeg, cloves, ginger and allspice. It's marketed by the leading spice companies and is available nationwide.

116 Calories; 2g Fat (14% CFF); 14g Protein; 12g Carbohydrate; 34mg Cholesterol; 409mg Sodium

Refried Bean Dip

Serves: 4   Preparation Time: 0:06

Amount	Measure	Ingredient — Preparation Method
1	cup	fat free refried beans
2	tablespoons	sweet red peppers — minced
2	tablespoons	raisins — minced
2	tablespoons	onions — minced
$\frac{1}{4}$	teaspoon	curry powder

Combine all ingredients. Microwave on high for 1 minute. Stir, serve with corn chips or crisp vegetables.

NOTES: This is a nice topping for individual nachos: put on chips, add cheese and heat.

93 Calories; <1g Fat (2% CFF); 4g Protein; 19g Carbohydrate; 0mg Cholesterol; 243mg Sodium

Grecian Sunset Appetizers

Serves: 8   Preparation Time: 0:40

Amount	Measure	Ingredient — Preparation Method
½	cup	sun-dried tomatoes — chopped
¼	cup	white wine
¼	cup	parsley sprigs — packed
⅓	cup	yellow peppers — chopped
¼	cup	sweet red peppers — chopped
¼	cup	reduced fat feta cheese — crumbled
2	tablespoons	kalamata olives — pitted
1	egg	
¼	cup	low fat cottage cheese

Preheat oven to 375°. Lightly coat 16 mini muffin cups with vegetable cooking spray.

Soak the sun-dried tomatoes in the wine, set aside. Put the remaining ingredients in a food processor bowl fitted with a chopping blade, pulse 5 times. Stop, scrape the sides of the bowl, add the tomatoes and wine, pulse 5 more times or until blended. Put a tablespoon of batter into each muffin cup.

Bake for 25-30 minutes or until firm and lightly browned. Remove from the muffin cups. Cool for a few minutes on a wire rack. Serve warm.

NOTES: There are no meek flavors here! Best served with a glass of good white wine.

---

66 Calories; 3g Fat (48% CFF); 5g Protein; 3g Carbohydrate; 32mg Cholesterol; 353mg Sodium

Smokin' Guacamole

Serves: 4   Preparation Time: 0:10

Amount	Measure	Ingredient — Preparation Method
1	medium	avocado — peeled, pitted
1	tablespoon	low fat mayonnaise
$\frac{1}{2}$	cup	salsa — prepared
$\frac{1}{4}$	cup	onions — minced
2	tablespoons	lemon juice
4	drops	hot pepper sauce

Using a food processor fitted with a chopping blade, blend all ingredients until smooth. Adjust seasonings. Makes about 1 cup.

NOTES: To store, press a piece of waxed paper directly on top of the guacamole to seal out air. Exposure to air is what turns avocado products brown. Contrary to popular belief, putting the pit of the avocado in the dip will not help to keep it green — except exactly where the pit lies!

100 Calories; 8g Fat (66% CFF); 2g Protein; 8g Carbohydrate; 0mg Cholesterol; 127mg Sodium

Peanut Butter Chicken Kabobs

Serves: 12   Preparation Time: 0:25

Amount	Measure	Ingredient — Preparation Method
$\frac{1}{3}$	cup	chunky peanut butter
3	tablespoons	soy sauce
2	tablespoons	cooking sherry
1	pound	chicken breast — boneless/skinless

Preheat grill or broiler. Lightly coat a broiler pan (if applicable) with vegetable cooking spray.

Soak 24 medium-sized bamboo skewers in water.

In a large bowl blend the first 3 ingredients. Cut chicken in 24 thin strips, coat with the mixture then thread onto skewers.

Grill or broil for 3-4 minutes on each side or until the chicken is no longer pink inside.

NOTES: Chicken cuts much easier when it's slightly frozen.

Soak the bamboo skewers in water for 30 minutes before using so they don't char during grilling.

92 Calories; 5g Fat (45% CFF); 10g Protein; 2g Carbohydrate; 23mg Cholesterol; 312mg Sodium

Hummus Wild Things

Serves: 12   Preparation Time: 0:20

Amount	Measure	Ingredient — Preparation Method
15	ounces	chickpeas, canned
2	tablespoons	lemon juice
2	teaspoons	garlic — minced
$\frac{1}{4}$	teaspoon	ground cumin
$\frac{1}{2}$	teaspoon	salt free seasoning
2	tablespoons	fresh cilantro — chopped
$\frac{1}{4}$	cup	red onions — chopped
1	medium	sweet red pepper — cut in wedges
1	medium	green pepper — cut in wedges
$\frac{1}{4}$	pound	jicama — peeled, cut thin
1	small	cucumber — sliced
$\frac{1}{4}$	cup	alfalfa sprouts

Drain chickpeas, reserving the liquid. Place the chickpeas in the bowl of a food processor fitted with a chopping blade. Add $\frac{1}{2}$ cup of the reserved liquid, blend until smooth. Add the lemon juice, garlic, cumin, seasoning, cilantro and onion. Blend until smooth.

Place the peppers, jicama and cucumber on a serving plate. Drop a teaspoonful of hummus onto each one and top with alfalfa sprouts. Serve chilled.

NOTES: To serve this appetizer right away, just start with pre-chilled ingredients.

59 Calories; 1g Fat (8% CFF); 2g Protein; 12g Carbohydrate; 0mg Cholesterol; 108mg Sodium

Library Resource Center
Renton Technical College
3000 N.E. 4th St.
Renton, WA 98056

Spinach Sticks

Serves: 12   Preparation Time: 0:50

Amount	Measure	Ingredient — Preparation Method
2	tablespoons	cornmeal
16	ounces	frozen chopped spinach — thawed, squeezed
$\frac{1}{4}$	cup	onions — minced
$\frac{1}{4}$	cup	sweet red pepper — minced
1	cup	bread stuffing — crushed
1	tablespoon	canola oil
$\frac{1}{4}$	cup	parmesan cheese — grated
4		egg whites — beaten
$\frac{1}{2}$	teaspoon	garlic powder
$\frac{1}{8}$	teaspoon	nutmeg
$\frac{3}{4}$	cup	bread stuffing — crushed fine
$\frac{1}{4}$	cup	sesame seeds

Preheat oven 350°. Sprinkle cornmeal evenly on a jelly roll pan, put aside.

In a large bowl combine everything except the last $\frac{3}{4}$ cup of crushed stuffing and the sesame seeds. Stir into a stiff dough and form one tablespoonful into a stick about 2" long. Repeat until the mixture is used up.

Mix the remaining crushed stuffing and sesame seeds together. Coat each stick in the mixture and place on the pan.

Bake for 15-20 minutes or until golden brown. Makes 24.

NOTES: These freeze well if stored between layers of waxed paper prior to baking. No need to thaw first, just add an extra 2 or 3 minutes to the baking time.

Don't let your guests struggle with spinach strings. Chop the spinach fine for an easy to eat appetizer.

A jelly roll pan is a large flat baking sheet with $\frac{1}{2}$" high sides. It's similar to a cookie sheet but more useful because it keeps foods from spilling off while baking.

109 Calories; 6g Fat (46% CFF); 5g Protein; 10g Carbohydrate; 1mg Cholesterol; 236mg Sodium

Cheryl Mochau

SAUCES, DIPS AND MARINADES

Cheryl Mochau

Mustard Dill Sauce

Serves: 4   Preparation Time: 0:05

Amount	Measure	Ingredient — Preparation Method
1	tablespoon	sugar
2	tablespoons	red wine vinegar
1	teaspoon	olive oil
5	tablespoons	Dijon mustard
1/4	teaspoon	dried dill weed
1/8	teaspoon	black pepper

Using a medium bowl, whisk the sugar and vinegar together until the sugar dissolves. Pour the oil in a thin stream while whisking briskly, add the mustard, dill and pepper. Reserve half to use as a sauce over cooked chicken, turkey, beef or fish and the remaining half for coating foods before cooking.

NOTES: Try whole seed Dijon mustard for a more robust flavor.

If you have fresh dill, substitute 1 tablespoon of it chopped for the dried dill. Fresh dill makes a glorious garnish!

37 Calories; 2g Fat (44% CFF); 1g Protein; 5g Carbohydrate; 0mg Cholesterol; 235mg Sodium

Tomato-Basil Yogurt Sauce

Serves: 4   Preparation Time: 0:10

Amount	Measure	Ingredient — Preparation Method
1	medium	tomato — peeled, chopped
2	tablespoons	fresh basil — chopped
1	tablespoon	sugar
1 ½	tablespoons	red wine vinegar
⅛	teaspoon	black pepper
¼	teaspoon	onion powder
8	ounces	plain low fat yogurt

Drain and discard the liquid from the tomato. Combine the tomato pulp with the remaining ingredients, chill. Serve chilled over cooked fish, chicken or as a vegetable dip.

NOTES: Peel the tomato into one long strip and roll to make a tomato rose for garnish.

Try a mixture of yellow and red tomatoes for brighter color and save a cluster of basil leaves for garnish.

56 Calories; 1g Fat (15% CFF); 3g Protein; 9g Carbohydrate; 3mg Cholesterol; 43mg Sodium

Creamy Caper Sauce

Serves: 2   Preparation Time: 0:05

Amount	Measure	Ingredient — Preparation Method
¼	teaspoon	garlic powder
¼	teaspoon	onion powder
1	teaspoon	lemon juice
2	tablespoons	light sour cream
1 ½	teaspoons	capers — drained

Combine all ingredients. Chill until ready to use. Serve as a topping for cooked fish, chicken or vegetables.

NOTES: Capers are the dried and pickled flower buds of a native Mediterranean shrub. They have a pungent, bitter taste and are best used in small amounts to enhance other foods.

11 Calories; 1g Fat (33% CFF); 0g Protein; 1g Carbohydrate; 1mg Cholesterol; 236mg Sodium

Orange Horseradish Dip

Serves: 6   Preparation Time: 0:05

Amount	Measure	Ingredient — Preparation Method
1	cup	light sour cream
3	tablespoons	orange marmalade
2	teaspoons	prepared white horseradish
1	teaspoon	orange peel — grated

Combine all ingredients. Chill until ready to use.

NOTES: A similar version of this recipe was presented to me by one of my clients. It became one of our favorites after we changed from non fat sour cream to light sour cream and eliminated honey and ground white pepper. We found this to be perfect for everything from a dip for pretzels and fruit to a sauce for chicken salads and grilled fish.

27 Calories; 1g Fat (3% CFF); 0g Protein; 7g Carbohydrate; 0mg Cholesterol; 8mg Sodium

Valerie's Teriyaki Marinade

Serves: 4   Preparation Time: 0:05

Amount	Measure	Ingredient — Preparation Method
¼	cup	brown sugar — packed
¼	cup	low sodium soy sauce
2	tablespoons	lemon juice
1	tablespoon	canola oil
¼	teaspoon	ground ginger
½	teaspoon	garlic — minced

Combine all ingredients. Marinate chicken, turkey, beef, fish or vegetables for 3 hours or more in the refrigerator. Rev up the grill!

NOTES: This delicious recipe was found in a Good Housekeeping magazine and is good for just about any method of cooking — not just grilling. See the 'So Fast Salad' recipe for an example conversion.

94 Calories; 3g Fat (31% CFF); 1g Protein; 16g Carbohydrate; 0mg Cholesterol; 605mg Sodium

Cheryl Mochau

SOUPS

Cheryl Mochau

Carrot & Ginger Soup

Serves: 8   Preparation Time: 1:20

Amount	Measure	Ingredient — Preparation Method
7	cups	low sodium chicken broth
1	cup	onions — chopped
1/4	cup	ginger root — peeled, minced
2	tablespoons	garlic — minced
1/2	teaspoon	curry powder
2	pounds	carrots — peeled, chopped
1	cup	white wine
2	tablespoons	lemon juice
		salt & pepper — to taste
1	tablespoon	fresh parsley — chopped

Boil ½ cup of broth in a large pot. Add the onion, ginger root and curry, reduce heat to medium, stir for 8 minutes until the onion is softened, adding more broth if needed. Raise the temperature to high, add the remaining broth and carrots. Cover, bring to a boil, reduce the heat and simmer for 20 minutes until the carrots are tender, stirring occasionally. Add the wine, lemon juice, salt and pepper. Simmer for 5 minutes more. Mash the carrots first, then using a hand-held electric blender or wire whisk, blend until smooth. Serve hot or chilled. Garnish with parsley.

NOTES: A hand-held electric blender is my tool of choice for pureeing this soup right in the pot, because it maneuvers easily in the pot and leaves the soup smooth with very little fuss. However, the molten liquid requires respect, so use caution!

69 Calories; 1g Fat (24% CFF); 1g Protein; 6g Carbohydrate; 0mg Cholesterol; 613mg Sodium

Eileen's Corn Soup

Serves: 6   Preparation Time: 0:25

Amount	Measure	Ingredient — Preparation Method
4	cups	vegetable broth
1	cup	onions — chopped
1	cup	sweet potato — diced small
½	cup	sweet red pepper — chopped
1 ¼	cups	corn kernels
2	teaspoons	chili powder
1		lime — sliced thin
2	tablespoons	fresh cilantro leaves — chopped

In a 2-quart saucepan bring the vegetable broth to a boil. Add everything except the cilantro and boil gently for 10 minutes. Remove from the heat, stir in the cilantro. Serve hot, leaving the lime slices as garnish. Makes 6 servings (½ cup each).

NOTES: When storing leftovers, remove the lime slices to avoid turning the soup bitter.

If fresh cilantro is not available, substitute 2 teaspoons of dried cilantro.

Cilantro, otherwise known as coriander leaves or Chinese parsley, has a distinctive, pungent odor and taste. When blended with the strong flavors of Mexican, Asian and Indian cooking, cilantro adds character and depth with its fragrant, green, lacy leaves. Coriander seeds also come from this ancient plant.

182 Calories; 3g Fat (14% CFF); 6g Protein; 35g Carbohydrate; 2mg Cholesterol; 1115mg Sodium

Yellow Split Pea Soup

Serves: 4   Preparation Time: 1:25

Amount	Measure	Ingredient — Preparation Method
1	cup	yellow split peas, dried — rinsed, drained
4	cups	low sodium chicken broth
1	teaspoon	garlic — minced
$\frac{1}{2}$	cup	onions — minced
$\frac{1}{4}$	cup	celery — minced
$\frac{1}{4}$	cup	carrots — minced
1	small	bay leaf
$\frac{1}{8}$	teaspoon	rosemary — crumbled
$\frac{1}{4}$	teaspoon	salt
$\frac{1}{8}$	teaspoon	black pepper
1	tablespoon	lemon juice

Pick any stones or debris from the peas.

Using a 4-quart covered saucepan, bring the broth to a boil, add the peas, garlic and onion. Boil rapidly for 2 minutes, then shut off the heat and let stand for 30 minutes.

Add the remaining ingredients — except for the lemon juice, bring back to a boil, reduce the heat to medium-low and boil gently uncovered for 40 minutes. Remove from the heat, discard the bay leaf, and stir in the lemon juice.

For a smooth consistency, puree the soup with a blender or wire whisk.

NOTES: Yellow split peas have a slightly sweeter taste than green split peas.

If the soup is too thin, do not despair! Pea soup thickens as it cools. If it's too thick, just add water and stir.

228 Calories; 2g Fat (7% CFF); 13g Protein; 39g Carbohydrate; 0mg Cholesterol; 841mg Sodium

Fennel & Orzo Soup

Serves: 4   Preparation Time: 0:30

Amount	Measure	Ingredient — Preparation Method
3	cups	low sodium chicken broth
$\frac{1}{3}$	cup	orzo
$\frac{1}{2}$	teaspoon	garlic — minced
$\frac{1}{4}$	cup	carrot — peeled, chopped
$\frac{1}{2}$	cup	turnip — peeled, cubed
$\frac{1}{2}$	cup	fennel bulb — chopped
$\frac{1}{4}$	teaspoon	caraway seed
$\frac{1}{8}$	teaspoon	black pepper

Using a 2-quart saucepan over high heat, bring the broth to a boil. Add the remaining ingredients, reduce the heat to medium, boil gently for 10-12 minutes. Makes 4 servings ($\frac{1}{2}$ cup each).

NOTES: This mildly flavored soup is perfect for a light lunch.

Fennel bulbs are sold in the produce section of major grocery stores. Choose a compact bulb with feathery greens that are also useful for garnishes and salads.

84 Calories; 1g Fat (2% CFF); 10g Protein; 11g Carbohydrate; 0mg Cholesterol; 420mg Sodium

Wild Mushroom Soup

Serves: 4   Preparation Time: 0:30

Amount	Measure	Ingredient — Preparation Method
1	pound	assorted mushrooms — cleaned, sliced
$\frac{1}{2}$	cup	onions — minced
1	tablespoon	flour
2	cups	low sodium beef broth
10	ounces	beef consommé
2	tablespoons	cognac
2	tablespoons	dry sherry
$\frac{1}{8}$	teaspoon	black peppercorns — ground
$\frac{1}{4}$	teaspoon	dried thyme — crushed

Lightly coat a 2-quart saucepan with vegetable cooking spray. Sauté the mushrooms and onions over medium-high heat for 5 minutes. Sprinkle with flour and stir to coat. Quickly add $\frac{1}{2}$ cup of the broth, stirring until the flour is smooth. Add the remaining broth and consommé, cover, bring almost to a boil, reduce heat, and simmer for 15 minutes. Add the remaining ingredients, cook for one minute. Makes about 4 cups.

NOTES: Choose from morel, shitake, wood ear, cepe, chanterelle and common cultivated mushrooms available at supermarkets nationwide.

106 Calories; 1g Fat (6% CFF); 11g Protein; 10g Carbohydrate; 0mg Cholesterol; 635mg Sodium

Snappy Vegetable Soup

Serves: 8   Preparation Time: 0:35

Amount	Measure	Ingredient — Preparation Method
4	cups	low sodium chicken broth
½	cup	onions — chopped
1	teaspoon	garlic — minced
¼	cup	green pepper — chopped
¼	cup	carrots — chopped
2	cups	tomatoes — peeled, diced
8	ounces	garbanzo beans, canned — rinsed, drained
1	teaspoon	Italian seasoning — dried
¼	teaspoon	thyme
⅛	teaspoon	black pepper
¼	cup	balsamic vinegar
3	tablespoons	soy sauce
2	tablespoons	Worcestershire sauce
2	teaspoons	lemon juice
⅓	cup	orzo

In a 4-quart saucepan over medium-high heat bring the broth to a boil. Add the onions, garlic, green pepper, carrots and tomatoes, boil gently for 5 minutes. Add the remaining ingredients, reduce the heat, simmer for 10 minutes or until the orzo is tender.

NOTES: Put any of your favorite vegetables into this versatile soup.

99 Calories; 1g Fat (4% CFF); 8g Protein; 16g Carbohydrate; 0mg Cholesterol; 772mg Sodium

Onion Soup

Serves: 6   Preparation Time: 0:40

Amount	Measure	Ingredient — Preparation Method
1	tablespoon	olive oil
2	cups	onions — chopped
1	tablespoon	flour
2	cups	low sodium beef broth
2	cups	low sodium chicken broth
$\frac{1}{2}$	cup	white wine
2	tablespoons	cooking sherry
$\frac{1}{8}$	teaspoon	black pepper
4	slices	stale bread
2	tablespoons	parmesan cheese — grated
2	tablespoons	mozzarella cheese — shredded

Using a 2-quart saucepan, warm the oil over medium-high heat. Add the onions, stir until dark brown, about 15 minutes. Sprinkle the flour over the onions, stir well to coat then quickly pour one cup of the broth in the pan, stirring until lump free. Add the remaining broth, cover, bring to a boil, then immediately reduce heat and simmer for 10 minutes. Add the wine and pepper, simmer for one minute. Ladle into soup bowls.

Meanwhile, make the croutons by trimming the bread to fit the soup bowls. Sprinkle with the cheeses. Place in a toaster oven, toast for 1-2 minutes or until the cheese melts and the bread is lightly browned. To serve, float a crouton on top of each bowl of hot soup.

NOTES: The combinations of beef and chicken broth and two kinds of wine make this a full bodied soup that is fast and easy to prepare.

158 Calories; 4g Fat (25% CFF); 11g Protein; 16g Carbohydrate; 4mg Cholesterol; 478mg Sodium

Cheryl Mochau

SALADS

Cheryl Mochau

Crabmeat Salad

Serves: 4   Preparation Time: 0:15

Amount	Measure	Ingredient — Preparation Method
8	ounces	crabmeat — rinsed, picked clean
2	tablespoons	sweet red pepper — minced
2	tablespoons	celery — minced fine
2	tablespoons	low fat mayonnaise
2	tablespoons	light sour cream
1 ½	teaspoons	lemon juice
⅛	teaspoon	fennel seed — crushed, chopped
¼	teaspoon	seasoned salt
⅛	teaspoon	black pepper
8	ounces	lettuce — rinsed, dried
½		lemon — cut in 4 wedges

Squeeze the crabmeat dry. In a separate bowl mix the next 8 ingredients. Fold in the crabmeat. Serve chilled on a bed of greens with lemon wedges for garnish.

NOTES: Use fresh or frozen crabmeat and try mesclun salad greens instead of just lettuce for a nice presentation.

76 Calories; 1g Fat (16% CFF); 11g Protein; 6g Carbohydrate; 45mg Cholesterol; 330mg Sodium

Chicken Caesar Salad

Serves: 4   Preparation Time: 0:20

Amount	Measure	Ingredient — Preparation Method
12	ounces	chicken breast — boneless/skinless
$\frac{1}{4}$	teaspoon	onion powder
$\frac{1}{8}$	teaspoon	garlic powder
$\frac{1}{8}$	teaspoon	dried thyme
4	ounces	low fat Caesar salad dressing
12	ounces	romaine lettuce leaves — washed, dried
$\frac{1}{4}$	cup	red onions — minced
3	tablespoons	parmesan cheese — grated
1	cup	croutons
1	teaspoon	freshly ground black pepper

Coat a skillet with vegetable cooking spray and place over medium heat.

Season the chicken with onion powder, garlic powder and thyme. Sauté for 7 minutes on each side or until no longer pink inside. Cut the cooked chicken into strips, keep warm.

Meanwhile, chop the lettuce, toss with the red onion, dressing and cheese. Place equal portions of the lettuce mixture on serving plates, top with the cooked chicken, croutons and freshly ground black pepper.

NOTES: If preparing ahead, store the cooked chicken in the refrigerator separately from the lettuce part of the salad. Reheat the chicken for 1-2 minutes in the microwave before placing it on top of the lettuce and adding the croutons and black pepper.

207 Calories; 6g Fat (26% CFF); 23g Protein; 14g Carbohydrate; 59mg Cholesterol; 485mg Sodium

Toaster Oven Croutons

Serves: 4   Preparation Time: 0:10

Amount	Measure	Ingredient — Preparation Method
2	slices	stale bread
10	shots	margarine spray
1	tablespoon	salt free seasoning
1	tablespoon	parmesan cheese — grated

Cut the bread into cubes, place in a bowl, spray with margarine, sprinkle with seasoning and cheese, toss to coat. Place on the toaster oven baking tray, toast until medium brown on all sides, turning as needed.

NOTES: Use just enough of the margarine spray to moisten the bread to hold the seasonings.

39 Calories; 1g Fat (17% CFF); 2g Protein; 8g Carbohydrate; 1mg Cholesterol; 121mg Sodium

Tuna-Jicama Salad

Serves: 4   Preparation Time: 0:15

Amount	Measure	Ingredient — Preparation Method
¼	cup	red wine vinegar
1	tablespoon	sugar
2	tablespoons	soy sauce
½	teaspoon	ground ginger
1	teaspoon	canola oil
½	pound	jicama — peeled
1		scallion — thinly sliced
12	ounces	tuna in water, canned — squeezed dry
8	ounces	green leaf lettuce — washed, dried

In a small bowl combine the vinegar, sugar, soy sauce, ground ginger and oil. Set aside.

Slice the jicama into very thin sticks about ½" long. Mix with the scallion and tuna. Add the vinegar mixture, toss to combine. Serve on a bed of torn lettuce leaves.

NOTES: Jicama resembles a potato with its firm, thin, brown skin. The crispy flesh inside is white, similar to a water chestnut. Jicama may be used raw in salads or cooked as a vegetable.

548 Calories; 5g Fat (8% CFF); 108g Protein; 12g Carbohydrate; 125mg Cholesterol; 1932mg Sodium

So Fast Salad

Serves: 4   Preparation Time: 0:06

Amount	Measure	Ingredient — Preparation Method
¼	cup	brown sugar — packed
¼	cup	low sodium soy sauce
2	tablespoons	lemon juice
1	tablespoon	canola oil
¼	teaspoon	ground ginger
½	teaspoon	garlic — minced
2	tablespoons	raisins
1	pound	broccoli stalks, shredded

In a large bowl combine everything except the broccoli stalks. Stir until the sugar dissolves. Add the broccoli stalks, toss to coat. Serve chilled.

NOTES: Shredded broccoli stalks, sometimes called broccoli hearts, are available in ready-to-use packages in the produce section of most large grocery stores. If you can't find them, shred your own stalks or substitute shredded cabbage.

138 Calories; 3g Fat (22% CFF); 2g Protein; 25g Carbohydrate; 0mg Cholesterol; 666mg Sodium

Cheryl Mochau

POULTRY ENTREES

Cheryl Mochau

Chicken Divan

Serves: 4   Preparation Time: 0:35

Amount	Measure	Ingredient — Preparation Method
12	ounces	chicken breast — boneless/skinless
10	ounces	broccoli, frozen — thawed
¼	cup	sweet red pepper — chopped
10	ounces	fat free cream of chicken soup, condensed
¼	cup	low fat mayonnaise
½	teaspoon	curry powder
1	cup	reduced fat cheddar cheese — shredded
¼	cup	seasoned breadcrumbs

Preheat oven to 350°. Lightly coat a 2-quart baking dish with vegetable cooking spray.

Boil the chicken until opaque inside, drain and cut bite sized. Squeeze the excess water from the broccoli. Place the chicken, broccoli and sweet red peppers in the bottom of the baking dish. In a separate bowl combine the soup, mayonnaise, curry powder and half of the cheese, pour over the chicken and vegetables. Sprinkle with the remaining cheese and breadcrumbs.

Bake for 20 minutes.

NOTES: Mrs. Williamson used to request this dish regularly. She was one of my very first cooking clients and we always enjoyed planning the weekly menus together.

299 Calories; 11g Fat (34% CFF); 31g Protein; 19g Carbohydrate; 77mg Cholesterol; 1160mg Sodium

Hot Salsa Chicken

Serves: 4   Preparation Time: 0:35

Amount	Measure	Ingredient — Preparation Method
12	ounces	chicken breast — boneless/skinless
1	whole	lime
½	teaspoon	onion powder
1	tablespoon	granulated sugar
1	teaspoon	cumin
1	teaspoon	Italian seasoning
2	teaspoons	minced roasted garlic
½	cup	salsa
4	tablespoons	reduced fat cheddar cheese — shredded
1		scallion — sliced thin

Preheat oven to 375°.

Trim, rinse and pat the chicken dry. Slice the lime into 4 thin rounds, reserve for garnish. Squeeze the juice of the remaining lime along with the onion powder, sugar, cumin, Italian seasoning and roasted garlic into a 2-quart baking dish. Coat the chicken in the mixture, lay each piece flat and spoon equal amounts of salsa on top. Sprinkle with cheese.

Cover, bake for 20-25 minutes or until the chicken is no longer pink inside. Garnish with thin slices of scallion and lime.

NOTES: Buying regular or roasted minced garlic in jars is a great timesaver. Purists may not think it worthy of refrigerator space, but the average person putting dinner on the table everyday can probably find a spot on the door for it.

150 Calories; 4g Fat (23% CFF); 21g Protein; 8g Carbohydrate; 56mg Cholesterol; 189mg Sodium

Mini Turkey Meatloaves

Serves: 4   Preparation Time: 0:50

Amount	Measure	Ingredient — Preparation Method
¼	cup	onions — minced
2	tablespoons	celery — minced
½	cup	fresh breadcrumbs — loosely packed
2	tablespoons	non fat milk
1		egg white
½	teaspoon	Worcestershire sauce
1	teaspoon	salt free seasoning
1	pound	ground turkey
¼	cup	ketchup — divided

Preheat oven to 375°. Lightly coat an 8" x 8" baking pan with vegetable cooking spray.

In a large bowl combine all ingredients, but use only half of the ketchup. Divide the mixture into 4 parts, form into small loaves and place in the pan. Coat the exterior of the loaves with the remaining ketchup.

Bake for about 35-40 minutes until the juices run clear and the loaves are crusty.

NOTES: Everyone gets plenty of crusty edges with these mini meatloaves.

---

212 Calories; 10g Fat (41% CFF); 22g Protein; 9g Carbohydrate; 90mg Cholesterol; 341mg Sodium

Spanish Rice Stuffed Peppers

Serves: 4   Preparation Time: 0:40

Amount	Measure	Ingredient — Preparation Method
1	cup	brown rice — cooked
2	large	bell peppers — cut in halves
8	ounces	ground chicken breast
½	cup	onions — chopped
1	cup	tomatoes, canned — with juice
2	tablespoons	ketchup
1	tablespoon	Worcestershire sauce
1	tablespoon	chili powder
½	teaspoon	dried basil
⅛	teaspoon	salt
⅛	teaspoon	black pepper
¼	cup	reduced fat cheddar cheese — shredded

Prepare 1 cup of rice according to the package directions (or use 1 cup of leftover rice).

Using a 2-quart saucepan, bring 5 cups of water to a boil. Cut the peppers through the stem in equal halves, discard the stem, seeds and ribs. Par-boil the peppers for 2 minutes in boiling water, remove with tongs and place upside-down to drain.

Preheat oven to 375°. Lightly coat a large skillet with vegetable cooking spray. Brown the turkey and onions over medium-high heat for 4 minutes, while breaking the meat into small pieces with a spatula. Add the cooked rice and remaining ingredients, except the cheese. Simmer for 10 minutes.

Fill the peppers with the mixture, place in an 8" x 8" x 2" baking dish, top with cheese. Bake for 10 minutes.

NOTES: Use a variety of colorful — red, yellow and green — peppers.

Evelyn Tribole published the original of this recipe in her Healthy Homestyle Cooking cookbook (Rodale Press, 1994). I've made it several times over the years and have hardly changed a thing. Everyone loves it!

305 Calories; 5g Fat (14% CFF); 19g Protein; 47g Carbohydrate; 39mg Cholesterol; 400mg Sodium

Chicken Enchiladas

Serves: 4   Preparation Time: 0:30

Amount	Measure	Ingredient — Preparation Method
1	pound	chicken breast — boneless/skinless
8	ounces	mushrooms — sliced
1	tablespoon	salt free seasoning — divided
$\frac{1}{4}$	cup	scallions — cut thin
2	tablespoons	black olives — sliced
$\frac{1}{3}$	cup	reduced fat cheddar cheese — shredded
8	medium	tortillas
15	ounces	tomato sauce
$\frac{1}{2}$	cup	water
$\frac{1}{4}$	teaspoon	garlic powder
1	tablespoon	chili powder
$\frac{1}{4}$	cup	cilantro — minced

Preheat oven to 400°.

Lightly coat a 9" x 13" x 2" baking dish with vegetable cooking spray, set aside. Lightly coat a skillet with vegetable cooking spray.

Warm the skillet over medium-high heat. Cut the chicken into bite-sized pieces. Sauté the chicken and mushrooms with 1 teaspoon of the salt free seasoning until no longer pink inside, about 7-8 minutes. Meanwhile, in a small bowl mix the remaining seasoning, scallions, olives and 2 tablespoons of the cheese.

Lay the tortillas on a flat surface, spoon equal amounts of the chicken mixture onto each one, roll and place seam-side down in the baking dish. Combine the tomato sauce, water, garlic and chili powders, spoon over all to the edges. Sprinkle with the remaining cheese and cilantro.

Cover, bake for 15 minutes or until piping hot inside.

NOTES: Check the labels for the fat content of different brands of tortillas, which can range from 0% to 8% fat per serving!

451 Calories; 9g Fat (18% CFF); 37g Protein; 54g Carbohydrate; 75mg Cholesterol; 1178mg Sodium

Chicken Chili

Serves: 8   Preparation Time: 1:00

Amount	Measure	Ingredient — Preparation Method
1	pound	ground chicken breast
1	cup	onions — chopped
2	teaspoons	garlic –– minced
½	cup	sweet red pepper — chopped
1	cup	green pepper — chopped
¼	teaspoon	dried thyme
¼	teaspoon	black pepper
1	whole	bay leaf
28	ounces	tomatoes, canned — chopped
3	ounces	tomato paste
14	ounces	kidney beans, canned — rinsed, drained
7	ounces	corn, canned — drained
¼	cup	red wine
2	tablespoons	chili powder — or to taste
2	tablespoons	chocolate chips — chopped
2	tablespoons	cilantro — chopped

Lightly coat a 6-quart pot with vegetable cooking spray and place over medium-high heat.

Brown the chicken, onions, garlic, peppers, thyme, pepper and bay leaf for 4-5 minutes. Add the remaining ingredients, reduce the heat to medium-low, simmer for 30 minutes.

Remove the bay leaf before serving.

NOTES: The small amount of chocolate adds a smoothness to the sauce, but probably isn't enough to be considered "a fix" (sorry Chocoholics). The better the quality of chocolate used, the smoother the result.

195 Calories; 3g Fat (16% CFF); 18g Protein; 24g Carbohydrate; 34mg Cholesterol; 527mg Sodium

Sweet & Sour Chicken

Serves: 4   Preparation Time: 0:30

Amount	Measure	Ingredient — Preparation Method
3	cups	cooked rice
12	ounces	chicken breast — boneless/skinless
1	cup	green pepper — cut bite-sized
1	cup	sweet red pepper — cut bite sized
1	cup	onions — cut bite sized
$\frac{1}{3}$	cup	light brown sugar — packed
3	tablespoons	cornstarch
20	ounces	pineapple chunks in juice — reserve juice
3	tablespoons	cider vinegar
2	tablespoons	ketchup
2	tablespoons	soy sauce

Prepare 3 cups of rice according to package directions, keep warm.

Lightly coat a large skillet with vegetable cooking spray. Cut the chicken into bite-sized pieces and sauté over medium-high heat for 4 minutes or until no longer pink inside. Prepare the vegetables, set aside.

Using a 2-quart saucepan, mix the brown sugar and cornstarch. Drain the pineapple juice into a measuring cup and add enough cold water to equal 2 ¼ cups of liquid, add to the cornstarch mixture. Whisk in the vinegar, ketchup and soy sauce. Cook over medium-high heat, stirring constantly until it thickens and bubbles. Gradually add the cooked chicken pieces, peppers, onions and pineapple chunks without stopping the boil. Stir for 2 minutes more. Remove from the heat. Serve over hot cooked rice.

NOTES: Have the rice simmering, the chicken sautéing and all vegetables cut to size before starting this wonderful sauce from the 50th anniversary issue of Betty Crocker's Creative Recipes with Bisquick® (1980).

503 Calories; 3g Fat (5% CFF); 25g Protein; 95g Carbohydrate; 51mg Cholesterol; 663mg Sodium

Plum Good Chicken

Serves: 4   Preparation Time: 0:45

Amount	Measure	Ingredient — Preparation Method
16	ounces	plums in juice, canned
1	teaspoon	lemon juice
2	tablespoons	soy sauce
1	teaspoon	onion powder
½	teaspoon	garlic powder
	pinch	cayenne pepper
⅛	teaspoon	black pepper
1	pound	chicken breast — boneless/skinless
1	tablespoon	cornstarch
¼	cup	cooking sherry
3		scallions — sliced thin

Preheat oven to 375°. Lightly coat an 8" x 8" baking pan with vegetable cooking spray.

Using a small sharp knife, cut a slit in each plum and remove each pit. Combine the plums and juice with the lemon juice, soy sauce, onion powder, garlic powder, cayenne and pepper in the pan. Coat the chicken in the mixture.

Cover, bake for 20 minutes, turn the chicken over and continue baking for another 10 minutes or until done.

Meanwhile, make a cornstarch slurry with the cornstarch and sherry, refrigerate until needed. Place the cooked chicken and plums on a serving platter, set aside and keep warm. Pour the pan juices into a small saucepan and bring to a slow boil. Whisk the chilled cornstarch slurry into the plum sauce stirring briskly over medium-high heat for 30 seconds or until slightly thickened and smooth. Pour the sauce over the chicken and plums, garnish with sliced scallions.

NOTES: *A cornstarch slurry is a mixture of cornstarch and a cold liquid, often water. It is mixed to form a thin paste to congeal and thicken hot liquids. Cornstarch on its own will form lumps, which is why it's best to mix it with liquid before pouring it into the food to be thickened. Cornstarch may also be sifted with dry foods, especially granular sugar, which helps to disperse it evenly.*

760 Calories; 3g Fat (3% CFF); 31g Protein; 159g Carbohydrate; 68mg Cholesterol; 589mg Sodium

Tomato-Feta Turkey

Serves: 4   Preparation Time: 0:35

Amount	Measure	Ingredient — Preparation Method
12	ounces	turkey breast cutlets — rinsed
1/8	teaspoon	pepper
1/2	teaspoon	garlic powder
4	ounces	honey ham — cut in 8 thin slices
1/4	cup	sun-dried tomatoes — chopped
1	whole	scallion — sliced thin
1/4	cup	reduced fat feta cheese — crumbled
2	teaspoons	fat free cottage cheese
1/4	cup	seasoned breadcrumbs

Preheat oven to 400°. Lightly coat an 8" x 8" pan with vegetable cooking spray.

Separate the turkey cutlets into 4 equal portions and lay on a flat surface. Season with the pepper and garlic powder. Put aside.

Overlap the ham slices on a flat surface to make 4 portions. In a small bowl mix together the sun-dried tomatoes, scallion, feta cheese and cottage cheese. Spoon equal amounts onto each ham portion, roll into 4 tight cylinders and place each one on a turkey cutlet. Roll each cutlet closed, coat with seasoned breadcrumbs and place seam side down on the pan.

Bake for 17-20 minutes or until the crumbs are lightly browned and the juices run clear.

NOTES: Hold the rolls together with toothpicks if you choose, otherwise, roll them tight and press down firmly in the baking pan to seal the seam.

The cottage cheese helps give the reduced fat feta cheese some creaminess without adding any extra fat.

241 Calories; 8g Fat (32% CFF); 31g Protein; 10g Carbohydrate; 77mg Cholesterol; 1060mg Sodium

Hay Nest Eggs

Serves: 2   Preparation Time: 0:30

Amount	Measure	Ingredient — Preparation Method
2 ½	cups	shoestring hash browns, frozen
½	cup	ham, extra lean — diced
2	whole	eggs
2	tablespoons	reduced fat cheddar cheese — shredded
1	teaspoon	parsley — chopped

Place a rack in the lower third of the oven. Preheat oven to 400°. Lightly coat a baking sheet with vegetable cooking spray.

Spread the hash browns in a single layer, bake for 10 minutes or until almost done. Separate them in half to form 2 "nests." Crack an egg into the center of each nest. Return to the oven for 2 minutes or until the egg white begins to set. Remove from the oven, sprinkle with the ham, cheese and parsley. Bake for an additional 2-4 minutes, or until the egg is done to your liking. Remove with a broad spatula.

NOTES: This recipe is perfect for 1 or 100 portions. Serve it at your next breakfast meeting and watch them wake up and smile!

220 Calories; 8g Fat (36% CFF); 15g Protein; 18g Carbohydrate; 237mg Cholesterol; 637mg Sodium

Mexican Cornbread Casserole

Serves: 8   Preparation Time: 1:05

Amount	Measure	Ingredient — Preparation Method
1	pound	ground turkey breast
1	cup	onions — chopped
¼	cup	water
1 ¼	ounces	taco seasoning mix — divided
1	cup	sweet red pepper — chopped
1	cup	green pepper — chopped
1	cup	onions — chopped
½	cup	celery — sliced thin
14	ounces	stewed tomatoes — drained
7	ounces	corn, canned — drained
14	ounces	kidney beans, canned — rinsed and drained
7	ounces	cornbread mix
2		egg whites
½	cup	non fat milk
1	tablespoon	sugar
4	ounces	fat free sour cream
1	cup	reduced fat cheddar cheese — shredded
½	teaspoon	chili powder

Lightly coat a large skillet with vegetable cooking spray. Sauté the turkey and onion until brown. Add the water and half of the taco flavoring mix. Cook over medium heat until all of the liquid is absorbed. Meanwhile, in a large bowl combine the peppers, onion, celery, tomatoes, corn and beans with the remainder of the taco flavoring mix, set aside. In a separate bowl combine the cornbread mix, egg whites, milk and sugar, set aside.

Preheat oven to 375°. Lightly coat a 9" x 13" x 2" baking dish with vegetable cooking spray.

Place the vegetables on the long sides of the baking dish and the meat mixture down the center. Leave 2" gaps at both ends of the pan and spoon the cornbread mixture there. Drop dollops of sour cream on the meat and vegetables, sprinkle with the cheese and chili powder. Cover the vegetable portion loosely with aluminum foil.

Bake for 35-40 minutes or until the cornbread is golden brown and dry when a cake tester inserted near the vegetables comes out clean.

NOTES: Ground turkey breast has a tendency to become dry because, unlike the less expensive ground turkey, no fat and skin are added.

354 Calories; 10g Fat (24% CFF); 24g Protein; 44g Carbohydrate; 42mg Cholesterol; 1099mg Sodium

Cheryl Mochau

BEEF AND PORK ENTREES

Cheryl Mochau

Lean Ham Casserole

Serves: 4   Preparation Time: 0:50

Amount	Measure	Ingredient — Preparation Method
6	ounces	pasta
2	tablespoons	cornstarch
$\frac{1}{4}$	cup	cold water
2	cups	fat free half and half
1	cup	reduced fat cheddar cheese — shredded
1	teaspoon	onion powder
2	tablespoons	celery — minced
$\frac{1}{8}$	teaspoon	black pepper
1	cup	extra lean ham — cubed
$\frac{1}{2}$	cup	sweet red pepper — chopped
1	tablespoon	fresh parsley — minced
2	tablespoons	breadcrumbs

Cook the pasta according to the directions on the package and drain. When done, preheat the oven to 375°. Lightly coat a 1-$\frac{1}{2}$-quart baking dish with vegetable cooking spray.

Blend the cornstarch and water in a small cup, refrigerate. Meanwhile, in a 2-quart saucepan over medium-high heat, bring the half and half nearly to a boil, in about 6 minutes, while stirring frequently. Add $\frac{3}{4}$ cup of cheese, onion powder, celery and black pepper. Stir the cornstarch and water mixture, whisk into the sauce until slightly thickened and lump free. Remove from the heat, fold in the pasta and ham. Spoon the mixture into the baking dish, level off, top with the chopped peppers, remaining cheese, parsley and breadcrumbs.

Bake at 375° for 30 minutes.

NOTES: Refrigerating the cornstarch and cold water mixture before adding it to the hot sauce will help the sauce to thicken successfully.

359 Calories; 9g Fat (22% CFF); 21g Protein; 47g Carbohydrate; 36mg Cholesterol; 827mg Sodium

Apricot - Onion Beef

Serves: 4   Preparation Time: 0:45

Amount	Measure	Ingredient — Preparation Method
12	ounces	flank steak
1	teaspoon	olive oil
$\frac{1}{2}$	teaspoon	onion powder
$\frac{1}{4}$	teaspoon	garlic powder
$\frac{1}{8}$	teaspoon	black pepper
1	envelope	onion soup mix — beef flavored
$\frac{1}{2}$	cup	apricot preserves
4		dried apricots — cut in half
$\frac{1}{2}$	cup	water

Warm a skillet over medium heat.

Rinse the beef and pat dry, coat with the oil, onion powder, garlic powder and pepper. Sauté the beef for 2 minutes on each side or until lightly browned. Meanwhile, mix the onion soup mix, preserves, apricots and water together and pour over the beef. Reduce the heat to low, cover tightly, let simmer for 35 minutes or until tender.

When done, remove the beef from the pan, let it rest for 5 minutes then cut in thin strips against the grain. Cover and keep warm. Meanwhile, raise the heat to medium-high and reduce the sauce to make a syrup. Spoon over the beef.

NOTES: Specializing in lower fat cooking, I don't get many requests for beef or pork dishes. This recipe seems to be a favorite when people are looking for something different. This recipe also works beautifully with — you guessed it — chicken or turkey.

597 Calories; 11g Fat (16% CFF); 23g Protein; 112g Carbohydrate; 44mg Cholesterol; 963mg Sodium

Slow Cooker Beef Brisket

Serves: 4   Preparation Time: 9:15

Amount	Measure	Ingredient — Preparation Method
1 ½	pounds	beef brisket, lean
1	tablespoon	garlic — minced
½	teaspoon	black pepper
⅛	teaspoon	curry powder
1	cup	onions — chopped
1	whole	bay leaf
½	cup	chopped tomatoes
½	cup	red wine

Buy the leanest meat possible and trim all visible fat from the beef. Rub the garlic, black pepper and curry powder into the beef.

Place a large skillet lightly coated with vegetable cooking spray over medium-high heat. Brown the beef for 2 minutes on each side.

Put the bay leaf and half of the onions in the bottom of the crock, place the beef on top and cover with the remaining ingredients. Cover tightly, turn the temperature to high. After one hour, reduce the temperature to low and simmer for 7-8 hours. When done, remove the meat to a cutting board. Let it rest for 10 minutes before cutting on an angle against the grain. Discard the bay leaf before serving.

NOTES: Do not refrigerate leftovers in the crock. The crock will take too long to cool down before it's safe to put it in the refrigerator and too long to come back up to a safe temperature before putting it back on the heating element. The result may be spoiled food and a cracked crock.

311 Calories; 13g Fat (40% CFF); 36g Protein; 6g Carbohydrate; 106mg Cholesterol; 157mg Sodium

Sandy's Beef Moussaka

Serves: 12   Preparation Time: 1:25

Amount	Measure	Ingredient — Preparation Method
3	medium	eggplants — sliced $\frac{1}{4}$" thick
1	cup	onions — chopped
1	tablespoon	garlic — minced
1 $\frac{1}{2}$	pounds	extra lean ground beef
$\frac{1}{2}$	teaspoon	dried oregano
1	teaspoon	dried basil
$\frac{1}{2}$	teaspoon	cinnamon
$\frac{1}{2}$	teaspoon	salt
$\frac{1}{2}$	teaspoon	pepper
2	cups	tomato sauce
2	tablespoons	breadcrumbs
1	tablespoon	olive oil
2	tablespoons	flour
$\frac{1}{4}$	teaspoon	salt
$\frac{1}{4}$	teaspoon	pepper
2	cups	non fat milk
2	whole	eggs — beaten
$\frac{1}{2}$	cup	parmesan cheese — grated
$\frac{1}{2}$	cup	reduced fat cheddar cheese — shredded

Preheat oven to broil. Lightly coat 2 cookie sheets with vegetable cooking spray.

Lay the eggplant slices in a single layer, season with pepper and broil until light brown on each side. Continue until all the eggplant is done, then reduce the oven temperature to 350°.

Meanwhile, warm a large skillet coated with vegetable cooking spray over medium-high heat. Brown the onion, garlic and meat. Drain off any fat. Season with oregano, basil, cinnamon, salt, pepper and tomato sauce. Stir in the breadcrumbs and set aside.

Cream sauce: In a 2-quart saucepan over medium heat warm the olive oil then sprinkle the flour, salt and pepper, leaving undisturbed until bubbly, about 1 minute. Whisk in the milk. Turn up the heat to medium-high and stir frequently until slightly thickened. Pour the hot cream sauce in a thin stream into the beaten eggs, whisking vigorously to avoid cooking the eggs. The mixture should be the consistency of loose pudding.

Assemble the moussaka by lightly coating a 9" x 13" x 2" baking dish with vegetable cooking spray. Using half of the eggplant, place 3 neat overlapping rows of the broiled eggplant in the bottom of the dish. Sprinkle 2 tablespoons of each cheese over the rows of eggplant and then spread all of the meat mixture evenly. Layer the remaining eggplant slices in 3 neat rows and press down firmly. Spread the cream sauce on top. Sprinkle with the remaining cheese. Bake for 40 minutes until the top is light brown and set.

NOTES: The fat content is lowered by using extra lean ground beef, a minimal amount of olive oil instead of butter, non fat milk and reduced fat cheddar cheese instead of whole milk products. To lower the fat grams even more, try lean ground chicken breast instead of the beef. The taste will be different, but still delicious!

256 Calories; 14g Fat (49% CFF); 18g Protein; 16g Carbohydrate; 82mg Cholesterol; 563mg Sodium

Osso Buco

Serves: 4   Preparation Time: 2:30

Amount	Measure	Ingredient — Preparation Method
1	tablespoon	olive oil
3	pounds	veal shank — cut in 4 pieces
$\frac{1}{4}$	cup	white flour
1	tablespoon	black pepper
2	teaspoons	garlic — minced
2	cups	onions — chopped
1	cup	tomatoes — peeled, chopped
$\frac{1}{4}$	cup	carrot — minced
$\frac{1}{2}$	cup	white wine
1	cup	beef consommé

Warm the oil in a large Dutch oven over medium heat. Dredge the veal shanks in flour and pepper, brown on all sides with the garlic and onions for about 15 minutes. Place the shanks cut side down then pour the remaining ingredients over them. Cover, simmer for 1 $\frac{1}{2}$ to 2 hours, turning occasionally. When done, the meat should be very tender. Remove from the pan, keep warm. Raise the heat to medium-high and reduce the liquid to thicken slightly. Serve with the juices and onions.

NOTES: The secret of great Osso Buco is having lots of marrow inside the bone and plenty of meat outside. Ask your butcher for the hind shanks and have them cut about 2" thick.

555 Calories; 14g Fat (25% CFF); 78g Protein; 20g Carbohydrate; 266mg Cholesterol; 744mg Sodium

FISH AND SEAFOOD ENTREES

Cheryl Mochau

Baked Tuna Steak & Paprika Sauce

Serves: 4   Preparation Time: 0:25

Amount	Measure	Ingredient — Preparation Method
½	teaspoon	paprika
¼	teaspoon	garlic powder
¼	teaspoon	onion powder
3	tablespoons	light sour cream
1	tablespoon	white wine
1		lemon — cut in 6 wedges
1	pound	tuna steak — cut in quarters
2	teaspoons	Dijon mustard
½	teaspoon	coarse black pepper
¼	cup	white wine

Sauce: Whisk together the paprika, garlic powder, onion powder, sour cream, wine and the juice of 1 lemon wedge in a small bowl, cover and refrigerate.

Preheat oven to 400°. Lightly coat an 8" x 8" baking dish with vegetable cooking spray.

Rinse the fish, pat dry, place in the baking dish and coat with the mustard, pepper, wine and the juice of 1 lemon wedge.

Cover, bake for 15-17 minutes or until the fish is opaque inside. Serve with the reserved sauce and remaining lemon wedges.

NOTES: Choose tuna steak that is firm to the touch, not at all sticky, with only the slightest fish odor.

---

190 Calories; 6g Fat (30% CFF); 28g Protein; 4g Carbohydrate; 44mg Cholesterol; 80mg Sodium

Fish Nets

Serves: 4 Preparation Time: 0:35

Amount	Measure	Ingredient — Preparation Method
5	cups	shoestring hash browns, frozen
¼	teaspoon	black pepper
2	cups	tomatoes — chopped, save juice
1	pound	cod fillets — cut in 4 pieces
¼	cup	fresh parsley — minced
1	teaspoon	dried thyme
1	tablespoon	sugar
12		kalamata olives — pitted and sliced
2	tablespoons	capers — with some juice
½	teaspoon	garlic powder
¼	cup	white wine
1		lemon — cut in 6 wedges

Preheat oven to 400°. Lightly coat a cookie sheet with vegetable cooking spray.

Spread the hashed browned potatoes in a single layer, season with pepper, and bake for 12 minutes or until brown and crispy. After the potatoes are done, pull apart 4 sections of "net material" about 4" in diameter, set aside and keep warm. Separate the remaining hash browns into 4 individual circles to form the bottoms of the "nets."

Using a large skillet over medium heat, warm ¼ cup of the tomato juice, add the fish pieces and remaining ingredients, except for 4 of the lemon wedges. Squeeze the juice of the 2 remaining lemon wedges on the fish. Turn the fish once after about 4 minutes. It will be done when it flakes easily with a fork at the thickest part, but remains intact. Lift the fish with a spatula and place one piece on each "net" bottom of hash browned potatoes. Turn the heat to medium-high, reduce the remaining tomato mixture until most of the liquid is evaporated. Spoon the sauce over the fish. Place the reserved "net material" on top. Garnish with the remaining lemon wedges.

NOTES: Just about any white fish will serve up nicely this way.

259 Calories; 4g Fat (15% CFF); 22g Protein; 30g Carbohydrate; 49mg Cholesterol; 307mg Sodium

Gina's Swordfish Raab

Serves: 4   Preparation Time: 0:25

Amount	Measure	Ingredient — Preparation Method
1	pound	swordfish steak — cut in quarters
1	whole	lemon — cut in 6 wedges
½	teaspoon	black pepper
1	teaspoon	olive oil
1 ½	cups	low sodium chicken broth
2	teaspoons	garlic — minced
½	cup	onions — chopped
½	cup	sweet red peppers — sliced thin
2	tablespoons	kalamata olives — pitted, sliced
5	cups	broccoli raab — rinsed, chopped

Preheat oven to broil. Lightly coat a broiler pan with vegetable cooking spray.

Season the fish with the juice of 2 lemon wedges, black pepper and oil. Broil for 4 minutes on each side or until done. Meanwhile, in a large pot bring the broth to a boil, add the garlic and onion, cook for one minute to soften. Add the remaining ingredients, cover, and cook over medium-high heat for 2-3 minutes until the broccoli raab is limp. Drain the liquid, arrange the broccoli raab on a serving platter, place the fish on top and garnish with the remaining lemon wedges.

NOTES: Broccoli raab (also known as broccoli di rape or broccoli rapini) is a member of the cabbage and turnip family. It looks similar to broccoli, but has several thin stalks instead of one thick one. It's sold in bunches and an average bunch is about 5 cups when chopped. A byproduct of the broccoli raab plant is the monounsaturated canola oil.

236 Calories; 8g Fat (30% CFF); 31g Protein; 13g Carbohydrate; 44mg Cholesterol; 447mg Sodium

South of the Border Salmon Filling

Serves: 4   Preparation Time: 0:15

Amount	Measure	Ingredient — Preparation Method
¼	cup	white wine
1	tablespoon	lemon juice
1	pound	salmon fillet — skinned
¼	cup	onions — minced
1 ¼	ounces	low sodium taco seasoning mix
⅓	cup	water
1	tablespoon	celery — minced

Warm a skillet over medium-high heat and put the wine, lemon juice, salmon and onion in. Sauté for 7 minutes or until the fish flakes easily. Mash the fish with a spatula, add the remaining ingredients and cook until the liquid is evaporated and the fish is completely cooked (about 3 minutes). Serve hot or cold.

NOTES: Serve in a pita pocket with lettuce and tomato or on a bed of lettuce for a simple salad.

172 Calories; 4g Fat (23% CFF); 23g Protein; 6g Carbohydrate; 59mg Cholesterol; 409mg Sodium

Spinach & Salmon Bake

Serves: 4   Preparation Time: 0:50

Amount	Measure	Ingredient — Preparation Method
1	pound	salmon fillet — skin removed
1	teaspoon	onion powder
1		lemon — cut in 6 wedges
1	cup	fat free cottage cheese
2		egg whites
3/4	teaspoon	low sodium chicken bouillon granules
1/4	cup	onions — minced
1/8	teaspoon	nutmeg
10	ounces	frozen spinach — thawed, squeezed
1/4	cup	sweet red peppers — minced
1/2	teaspoon	salt free seasoning
1/8	teaspoon	black pepper — or to taste
1/2	cup	Jarlsberg cheese — grated
3	tablespoons	parmesan cheese — grated
3	tablespoons	seasoned breadcrumbs

Preheat the oven to 400°. Lightly coat a 1-½-quart baking dish with vegetable cooking spray.

Season the salmon with the onion powder and the juice of 2 lemon wedges. Cover, bake for 10 minutes. Remove from the oven. Discard any dark spots on the fish, flake with a fork, spread evenly in the bottom of the baking dish. Reduce the oven temperature to 350°.

In a separate bowl combine the cottage cheese, egg whites, bouillon, onion, nutmeg, spinach, red peppers, seasoning and black pepper. Pour on top of the fish. Sprinkle with the cheeses and breadcrumbs.

Bake in a 350° oven for 30 minutes. Garnish with the remaining lemon wedges.

NOTES: Use a clear glass baking dish to show off these colorful layers.

Jarlsberg cheese is similar to Swiss cheese and is available in low fat form.

295 Calories; 10g Fat (29% CFF); 40g Protein; 14g Carbohydrate; 77mg Cholesterol; 704mg Sodium

Rice with Shrimp & Asparagus

Serves: 4   Preparation Time: 0:35

Amount	Measure	Ingredient — Preparation Method
3	cups	low sodium chicken broth
1/2	cup	onions — minced
1 1/2	cups	white rice
1	teaspoon	garlic — minced
1/2	cup	white wine
1	pound	asparagus — trimmed, sliced 1"
1/2	cup	sweet red pepper — sliced thin, 1" long
1	pound	shrimp — peeled, deveined
1	whole	lemon — cut in half
1/4	cup	parmesan cheese — grated

In a 2-quart saucepan bring the broth to boil. Add the onion and white rice, cover, and reduce to simmer for 20 minutes. Meanwhile, lightly coat a large skillet with vegetable cooking spray. Sauté the garlic over medium-high heat for 30 seconds, add half of the wine, bring to a boil, and add the asparagus and peppers, cook for 2 minutes. Push the vegetables to the coolest side of the skillet, pour in a bit more wine and add the shrimp. Cook briefly, just until pink on both sides then combine the shrimp and vegetables, adding any remaining wine. Remove from the heat.

Lightly coat a 2-quart baking dish with vegetable cooking spray. Spoon the rice in the bottom, pour the shrimp mixture evenly on top and squeeze the juice of half a lemon over all. Sprinkle with cheese. To garnish, arrange some of the asparagus tips and red pepper strips decoratively on top of the cheese.

Bake for about 15 minutes until the cheese melts. Cut the remaining lemon half into 4 wedges for garnish.

NOTES: Don't overcook the shrimp with the vegetables. They will cook more in the oven while the cheese melts.

485 Calories; 4g Fat (8% CFF); 40g Protein; 67g Carbohydrate; 176mg Cholesterol; 657mg Sodium

North Shore Scallops

Serves: 4   Preparation Time: 0:10

Amount	Measure	Ingredient — Preparation Method
1	pound	bay scallops
1	whole	lemon — cut in 6 wedges
1/4	cup	white wine
2	tablespoons	parsley — chopped
1/8	teaspoon	salt
1/8	teaspoon	black pepper
1	teaspoon	butter
4	sprigs	fresh parsley

Rinse the scallops under cold running water, drain. Using a large skillet over medium heat, add the juice of 2 lemon wedges, the wine and scallops. Within 1 or 2 minutes the scallops should begin to turn opaque underneath. Turn them over, season with the chopped parsley, salt and pepper, let simmer for another minute or until they begin to turn opaque inside. Remove to a serving dish immediately and keep warm (the trapped internal heat will continue to cook them slightly).

Raise the heat to medium-high. Add the butter and reduce the liquid in the skillet by half. Pour over the scallops. Garnish with the remaining lemon wedges and fresh parsley sprigs.

NOTES: *The seafood is unbelievably fresh on the North Shore of Boston. My friends at Rowand's Fishery were always helpful with fish selection and cooking tips.*

If you must watch your cholesterol closely, then substitute margarine for the butter.

---

137 Calories; 2g Fat (15% CFF); 20g Protein; 8g Carbohydrate; 40mg Cholesterol; 280mg Sodium

Tuna In a Pita

Serves: 4   Preparation Time: 0:15

Amount	Measure	Ingredient — Preparation Method
¼	cup	red wine vinegar
1	tablespoon	sugar
2	tablespoons	tamari soy sauce
½	teaspoon	ground ginger
1	teaspoon	lemon juice
1	tablespoon	low fat mayonnaise
12	ounces	tuna in water, canned — drained
1	cup	broccoli florets
1	cup	sweet red peppers — chopped
1	tablespoon	red onions — minced
2	tablespoons	water chestnuts — chopped
¼	pound	lettuce leaves
1	medium	tomato — sliced
4		pita bread — cut open

In a large bowl combine the vinegar, sugar, soy sauce, ginger, lemon juice and mayonnaise. Whisk to dissolve, set aside. Squeeze the tuna dry, add the broccoli, peppers, onion and water chestnuts. Mix well. Add the tuna mixture to the sauce, toss to combine. Serve in pita pockets with lettuce and tomato.

NOTES: Tamari soy sauce is made from fermented soy beans. It has a deep, rich flavor and nutrients that are revered in Asian cooking.

Save time. Buy pre-sliced water chestnuts and chop them.

317 Calories; 2g Fat (6% CFF); 30g Protein; 45g Carbohydrate; 26mg Cholesterol; 1156mg Sodium

VEGETABLE DISHES AND STARCHES

Cheryl Mochau

Tofu & Asparagus Pasta Bake

Serves: 4   Preparation Time: 0:50

Amount	Measure	Ingredient — Preparation Method
6	ounces	fat free egg noodles
1	pound	asparagus — trimmed, sliced
½	cup	sweet red pepper — cut in strips
1	cup	black beans — rinsed, drained
¼	cup	onions — chopped
8	ounces	tofu, medium — drained
11	ounces	fat free cream of celery soup, condensed
¼	cup	low fat mayonnaise
¼	teaspoon	curry powder
⅛	teaspoon	black pepper
¼	cup	seasoned breadcrumbs

Preheat the oven to 375°. Lightly coat a 2-quart baking dish with vegetable cooking spray, set aside.

Cook the egg noodles according to the directions. Two minutes before the noodles are done, add the asparagus and sweet red peppers, cover, bring back to a boil for 1 minute, drain. Meanwhile, in a medium bowl combine the remaining ingredients except for the breadcrumbs. Fold in the noodles and vegetables. Pour the mixture into the baking dish, top with breadcrumbs.

Bake for 30 minutes or until the top is lightly browned.

NOTES: Save time by parboiling the asparagus and peppers with the boiling noodles. This will give the vegetables a head start so they cook thoroughly in the casserole.

479 Calories; 7g Fat (13% CFF); 24g Protein; 81g Carbohydrate; 3mg Cholesterol; 868mg Sodium

Four Bean Vegetarian Chili

Serves: 8   Preparation Time: 0:50

Amount	Measure	Ingredient — Preparation Method
14	ounces	kidney beans, canned
14	ounces	black beans, canned
14	ounces	navy beans, canned
14	ounces	garbanzo beans, canned
7	ounces	corn, canned
1	tablespoon	canola oil
2	cups	onions — chopped
2	tablespoons	garlic — minced
1		bay leaf
8	ounces	mushrooms — sliced
1	cup	green pepper — chopped
28	ounces	tomatoes, canned — diced
6	ounces	tomato paste
3	tablespoons	black olives — sliced
1	tablespoon	oregano
2	tablespoons	chili powder — to taste

Rinse and drain the beans and corn, set aside. Warm the oil in a large pot over medium-high heat, add the onions, garlic, bay leaf, mushrooms and green pepper. Stir until the onions are lightly browned. Add the beans, corn, and remaining ingredients, cover, bring to a boil then immediately reduce the heat to simmer for 20 minutes. Adjust seasonings. Remove the bay leaf before serving.

NOTES: Using canned beans, corn and tomatoes makes this a super easy chili (just remember to recycle those cans!).

330 Calories; 4g Fat (11% CFF); 17g Protein; 61g Carbohydrate; 0mg Cholesterol; 975mg Sodium

Spinach & Feta Pasta

Serves: 4   Preparation Time: 0:35

Amount	Measure	Ingredient — Preparation Method
6	ounces	penne pasta
$\frac{1}{4}$	cup	red wine vinegar
1	teaspoon	olive oil
2	tablespoons	pine nuts (pignoli)
1	tablespoon	garlic — minced
4	ounces	fresh baby spinach — rinsed
1	cup	cherry tomatoes — cut in half
8	ounces	black beans, cooked — rinsed, drained
3	ounces	artichoke hearts, marinated — quartered
4		kalamata olives — pitted, sliced
1	cup	fat free cottage cheese
3	ounces	reduced fat feta cheese — crumbled
$\frac{1}{8}$	teaspoon	black pepper

Cook the pasta according to the directions and drain. In a large mixing bowl whisk the red wine vinegar and olive oil together, add the pasta and toss to coat. Set aside.

Lightly coat a large skillet with vegetable cooking spray and place over medium heat. Add the pine nuts and garlic, stirring until they begin to brown. Shake excess water from the spinach, add to the skillet and stir as the remaining water evaporates. Add the tomatoes, beans and artichoke hearts (including liquid), bring to a boil, reduce the heat and simmer for 3 minutes. Remove from the heat, fold in the remaining ingredients. Serve hot or cold.

NOTES: *Baby spinach is nice to work with because there are no thick stems to remove and the leaves are tender. It's sold prewashed and bagged in the produce section of major grocery stores. Be sure to rinse it for this recipe because the evaporating water plays a crucial role.*

422 Calories; 11g Fat (29% CFF); 22g Protein; 40g Carbohydrate; 10mg Cholesterol; 585mg Sodium

Oven Baked LaPenne

Serves: 6   Preparation Time: 0:50

Amount	Measure	Ingredient — Preparation Method
7	ounces	penne pasta
1	cup	onions — chopped
½	cup	green peppers — chopped
4	ounces	mushrooms — cleaned, sliced
2	teaspoons	garlic — minced
28	ounces	tomatoes, canned — chopped
6	ounces	tomato paste
2	cups	tomato sauce
1	teaspoon	sugar
½	cup	white wine
1	teaspoon	Italian seasoning
8	ounces	fat free ricotta cheese
4	ounces	part skim milk mozzarella cheese

Boil the pasta and drain. Meanwhile, sauté the onions, peppers, mushrooms and garlic over medium-high heat for 3 minutes. Add the tomatoes, paste, sauce, sugar and wine. Reduce heat to low, simmer for 5 minutes. Stir in the seasoning, remove from the heat, and combine with the cooked pasta.

Preheat oven to 375°. Lightly coat a 9" x 13" baking dish with vegetable cooking spray.

Spoon the mixture into the baking dish. Drop dollops of the ricotta cheese on top, press in slightly and sprinkle with the mozzarella cheese. Cover, bake for 30 minutes.

NOTES: Penne pasta is a tubular pasta that is similar to ziti, but is narrower and is cut on an angle.

For a crispier topping do not cover while baking.

322 Calories; 4g Fat (15% CFF); 17g Protein; 38g Carbohydrate; 14mg Cholesterol; 1056mg Sodium

Layered Vegetable Casserole

Serves: 4   Preparation Time: 1:00

Amount	Measure	Ingredient — Preparation Method
1	cup	instant rice — uncooked
4	ounces	mushrooms — sliced
1	cup	onions — chopped
½	cup	carrots — sliced
8	ounces	corn, canned — with juice
½	cup	green beans — sliced
½	cup	sweet red peppers — chopped
1	cup	garbanzo beans, canned — rinsed, drained
1	tablespoon	salt free seasoning
14	ounces	tomatoes, canned — with juice, chopped
3	ounces	reduced fat feta cheese — crumbled
½	cup	reduced fat cheddar cheese — shredded
1	teaspoon	sesame seeds

Preheat oven to 400°. Lightly coat a 2-quart baking dish with vegetable cooking spray.

Layer the ingredients in baking dish in the order they are listed. Cover tightly, bake for 40 minutes or until the vegetables are tender.

NOTES: The rice will absorb the vegetable juices, making it flavorful and moist.

335 Calories; 7g Fat (18% CFF); 16g Protein; 57g Carbohydrate; 18mg Cholesterol; 864mg Sodium

Vegetable Lasagna

Serves: 12   Preparation Time: 1:35

Amount	Measure	Ingredient — Preparation Method
1	cup	onions — chopped
1	cup	carrots — shredded
8	ounces	mushrooms — sliced
8	ounces	fresh spinach
32	ounces	tomato sauce
28	ounces	tomatoes, canned — chopped, drained
1	teaspoon	garlic — minced very fine
2	teaspoons	dried oregano — divided
16	ounces	tofu, medium — drained, crumbled
8	ounces	fat free cottage cheese
1	cup	part skim milk mozzarella cheese — shredded
3	tablespoons	parmesan cheese — shredded
9		lasagna noodles — uncooked

Lightly coat a large skillet with vegetable cooking spray. Over medium-high heat, sauté the onions, carrots and mushrooms until soft (about 8 minutes). Stir in the spinach until wilted, about 2-3 minutes.

In a large bowl combine the tomato sauce, tomatoes, garlic and half of the oregano. Set aside. In a separate bowl mash the tofu and blend with the cottage cheese, set aside.

Preheat the oven to 375°. Using a 10" x 15" x 2" nonreactive baking dish, assemble the lasagna by spreading one cup of the tomato mixture on the bottom of the dish and placing three noodles with equal space between them (they will absorb the liquids and expand). Layer one half of the vegetables and tofu mixture over the noodles then one third of the tomato sauce. Press down firmly, then repeat the layers finishing with 3 noodles on top covered completely by the remaining sauce. Cover tightly with foil. Bake for 45 minutes.

Uncover and sprinkle with the mozzarella and parmesan cheeses and the remaining oregano. Bake an additional 20 minutes. Remove from the oven. Let it sit for at least 15 minutes before cutting so the pasta may fully absorb the remaining liquids.

NOTES: The pasta will absorb the liquids and expand beyond the confines of a 9" x 13" baking dish. Trust me on this — use a larger baking dish!

If tofu isn't your thing, just replace it with low fat ricotta cheese.

368 Calories; 5g Fat (13% CFF); 20g Protein; 62g Carbohydrate; 7mg Cholesterol; 729mg Sodium

Hearty Lentil Stew

Serves: 4   Preparation Time: 0:55

Amount	Measure	Ingredient — Preparation Method
½	cup	lentils — rinsed, picked over
1	cup	potatoes — peeled, cubed
1	cup	baby carrots — cut lengthwise
1	cup	pearl onions — peeled
1	rib	celery — chopped
1	teaspoon	garlic — minced
2	cups	tomato juice
2	cups	low sodium chicken broth
2	teaspoons	chili powder
½	teaspoon	dried basil
½	teaspoon	dried oregano

Combine all ingredients in a large pot, bring to a boil, reduce heat and simmer for 40 minutes. Stir occasionally. Add a small amount of water if the broth gets too thick.

NOTES: When time is short, use frozen baby onions instead of fresh pearl onions and add a teaspoon of onion powder to boost the flavor.

204 Calories; 1g Fat (3% CFF); 15g Protein; 37g Carbohydrate; 0mg Cholesterol; 843mg Sodium

Spinach Casserole

Serves: 4   Preparation Time: 0:40

Amount	Measure	Ingredient — Preparation Method
10	ounces	frozen spinach — thawed, squeezed
½	cup	onions — chopped
½	cup	sweet red pepper — chopped
4		egg whites
1	cup	fat free half and half
1	cup	light ricotta cheese
⅛	teaspoon	black pepper
⅛	teaspoon	nutmeg

Preheat oven to 375°. Lightly coat an 8" x 8" x 2" baking dish with vegetable cooking spray.

Combine all ingredients in a large bowl. Pour into the prepared baking dish.

Bake for 30 minutes or until a tester inserted in the center comes out clean.

NOTES: A hint of nutmeg brings out the best in cooked spinach.

Fresh spinach can work well in this dish as long as it's blanched and squeezed dry before mixing in.

125 Calories; 3g Fat (21% CFF); 12g Protein; 12g Carbohydrate; 15mg Cholesterol; 193mg Sodium

Baked Stuffed Acorn Squash

Serves: 4   Preparation Time: 0:55

Amount	Measure	Ingredient — Preparation Method
2	small	acorn squash — cut in half
1	cup	apple — peeled, chopped
4	tablespoons	raisins
4	tablespoons	brown sugar
½	teaspoon	cinnamon
1	tablespoon	flour
½	teaspoon	vanilla powder

Preheat oven to 400°.

Scoop the seeds out of the squash and discard or roast with seasonings later. Set the squash halves upright in an 8" x 8" x 2" baking dish. Combine the remaining ingredients in a small bowl and spoon into each cavity. Pour 2 cups of hot water into the baking dish around the squash.

Cover tightly, bake for 40-50 minutes or until the squash is fork tender.

NOTES: For best results choose acorn squash that weigh less than 1 pound each.

195 Calories; 1g Fat (2% CFF); 2g Protein; 50g Carbohydrate; 0mg Cholesterol; 13mg Sodium

Caramelized Carrots

Serves: 4   Preparation Time: 0:15

Amount	Measure	Ingredient — Preparation Method
2	cups	baby carrots — rinsed
1	tablespoon	butter
¼	cup	brown sugar — packed
½	teaspoon	onion powder
¼	teaspoon	black pepper

Using a large skillet bring 2 cups of water to a boil. Add the carrots, cover, return to a boil for 4 minutes or until almost tender. Drain, do not rinse. Remove.

Reduce the temperature to medium, melt the butter in the skillet, and add the brown sugar and seasonings. Using a large flat spatula, scrape the mixture off the bottom of the pan as the bubbling liquid forms and the sugar completely dissolves. Add the carrots, coat with the syrup and continue cooking for another 2-3 minutes until the carrots are fork tender.

NOTES: Molten sugar will cause serious burns. Use extreme caution not to splash the mixture when making this recipe.

100 Calories; 3g Fat (26% CFF); 1g Protein; 19g Carbohydrate; 8mg Cholesterol; 67mg Sodium

Crispy Mixed Vegetables

Serves: 4   Preparation Time: 0:10

Amount	Measure	Ingredient — Preparation Method
½	cup	low sodium chicken broth
½	cup	onions — cut in thin strips
½	cup	baby carrots — cut lengthwise
½	cup	green beans — trimmed, cut ½"
¼	teaspoon	cornstarch
1	tablespoon	cold water
⅛	teaspoon	black pepper
½	cup	peas, frozen — thawed

In a 2-quart saucepan over high heat bring the broth to a boil. Add the onions and carrots, cover, bring back to a boil, then reduce the heat and simmer for 2 minutes. Add the green beans, stir for about one minute until they turn bright green. Meanwhile, mix the cornstarch and black pepper with the cold water in a small cup, pour into the broth and whisk to thicken slightly. Add the peas and stir to coat everything for 20-30 seconds. Remove from the heat while the vegetables are still crisp.

NOTES: The cornstarch, black pepper and water are mixed into the broth to make a very thin sauce that allows the seasonings to cling to the fresh vegetables.

38 Calories; 1g Fat (3% CFF); 3g Protein; 7g Carbohydrate; 0mg Cholesterol; 95mg Sodium

Green Beans Amandine

Serves: 4   Preparation Time: 0:10

Amount	Measure	Ingredient — Preparation Method
12	ounces	green beans — trimmed
1	tablespoon	butter
1	teaspoon	garlic — minced
2	tablespoons	sliced almonds
½	teaspoon	onion powder
½	teaspoon	seasoned salt

Using a 2-quart saucepan, bring ½ cup of water to a boil. Add the green beans, cover, bring back to a boil and cook for 1 minute. Drain and set aside.

Meanwhile, in a large skillet over medium-high heat, melt the butter, add the garlic, cook for 30 seconds then add the almonds and seasonings. Cook until the almonds are lightly browned (about 2 minutes), remove from the heat. Add the green beans, toss to coat. Serve hot.

NOTES: Substitute margarine for the butter if you are counting cholesterol content closely.

For best results use fresh green beans. Wash them first, then make neat piles, lining them up on a cutting board like a deck of cards, then trimming both ends evenly and efficiently with a couple of swift knife strokes.

---

80 Calories; 5g Fat (55% CFF); 3g Protein; 7g Carbohydrate; 8mg Cholesterol; 205mg Sodium

Cheryl Mochau

Roasted Medley of Vegetables

Serves: 4   Preparation Time: 0:50

Amount	Measure	Ingredient — Preparation Method
2	medium	parsnips — scrubbed, cubed
1	small	sweet potato — peeled, cubed
1	small	Vidalia onion — peeled, sliced
1	tablespoon	olive oil
1	tablespoon	salt free seasoning

Preheat oven to 400°. Lightly coat a jelly roll pan with vegetable cooking spray.

Place the vegetables in a mixing bowl, pour the oil and flavorings over all, and toss to coat. Spread the vegetables in a single layer on the pan.

Roast for 20 minutes, turn with a spatula, continue roasting for another 15-20 minutes or until the vegetables are fork-tender.

NOTES: Parsnips have a pale yellow skin and usually require nothing more than a quick scrub. However, they're occasionally encased in wax as a preservative and therefore must be peeled before using.

125 Calories; 4g Fat (25% CFF); 2g Protein; 24g Carbohydrate; 0mg Cholesterol; 12mg Sodium

Spinach Parm Patties

Serves: 4   Preparation Time: 0:40

Amount	Measure	Ingredient — Preparation Method
½	cup	onions — minced
10	ounces	frozen spinach — thawed, squeezed
1		egg white
¼	teaspoon	garlic powder
⅛	teaspoon	nutmeg
⅛	teaspoon	black pepper
4	tablespoons	light ricotta cheese
4	tablespoons	parmesan cheese — grated, divided
¼	cup	breadcrumbs
4	tablespoons	tomato sauce
⅛	teaspoon	oregano

Lightly coat an 8" x 8" baking pan with vegetable cooking spray, set aside.

Lightly coat a skillet with vegetable cooking spray. Sauté the onions until light brown. Meanwhile, mix together the spinach, egg white, garlic powder, nutmeg and pepper. Blend in the cooked onions. Divide the spinach mixture into 8 parts, flatten into patties.
Preheat the oven to 375°. Sprinkle the breadcrumbs on a flat surface and place the patties on the crumbs. Put one tablespoon of ricotta cheese and ½ tablespoon of the parmesan cheese on 4 of the patties. Top with the remaining patties, seal the edges with your fingers, coat with the breadcrumbs. Place in the baking pan. Smooth a tablespoon of tomato sauce on top of each patty, sprinkle with the remaining parmesan cheese and oregano.

Bake for 20-25 minutes or until lightly browned.

NOTES: These patties make a nice presentation when served with North Shore Scallops and Lauren's Rice Pilaf.

100 Calories; 3g Fat (25% CFF); 7g Protein; 12g Carbohydrate; 8mg Cholesterol; 324mg Sodium

Sweet Potato Tagine

Serves: 8   Preparation Time: 0:40

Amount	Measure	Ingredient — Preparation Method
4	cups	sweet potato – peeled, cubed
1	cup	green beans — cut 1" long
1	tablespoon	olive oil
1	tablespoon	curry powder
1	tablespoon	garlic — minced
1	cup	onions — chopped
2	teaspoons	low sodium chicken bouillon granules
$\frac{1}{4}$	cup	white wine
1	whole	bay leaf
2	tablespoons	raisins — chopped
$\frac{1}{4}$	cup	dried apricots — cut in half
2	cups	tomatoes — chopped
1	cup	black beans, cooked — rinsed, drained
2	tablespoons	sesame seeds — toasted

Using a 2-quart saucepan boil the sweet potatoes until fork-tender in just enough water to barely cover them. Remove with a slotted spoon, drain, and reserve. Bring the potato water back to a boil, add the green beans, and boil rapidly for 1 minute until they turn bright green. Remove with a slotted spoon, drain, and reserve. Save the potato water.

Using a large skillet over medium-high heat, sauté the oil and curry powder for 30 seconds, add the garlic, onion and $\frac{1}{4}$ cup of the potato water. Stir for 3 minutes, adding more potato water when it dries out, $\frac{1}{4}$ cup at a time. Add the bouillon, wine, bay leaf, raisins, dried apricots, tomatoes and black beans. Boil gently for 10 minutes, adding more of the potato water to keep the mixture at a sauce-like consistency. Fold in the reserved sweet potatoes and green beans. Remove from the heat, discard the bay leaf, spoon into a serving dish and sprinkle with toasted sesame seeds.

NOTES: Spread the sesame seeds on a small baking tray and pop them into the toaster oven set for light toast.

177 Calories; 4g Fat (17% CFF); 5g Protein; 33g Carbohydrate; 0mg Cholesterol; 166mg Sodium

Green Bean Bundles

Serves: 4   Preparation Time: 0:15

Amount	Measure	Ingredient — Preparation Method
4	long	scallions
1	teaspoon	olive oil
1	teaspoon	garlic — minced
2	tablespoons	balsamic vinegar
$\frac{1}{4}$	cup	low sodium chicken broth
8	ounces	fresh green beans — ends trimmed
$\frac{1}{8}$	teaspoon	black pepper

Choose the longest scallion shoots, rinse and lay flat on a plate, microwave for 15 seconds to soften. Let cool.

Using a heavy skillet over medium-high heat, warm the oil, add garlic and stir until light brown. Add the vinegar and broth. Bring to a boil. Add the beans and pepper, stirring constantly for 1-2 minutes, until they turn a deep shade of green but are still crisp. Remove from the heat immediately.

Lay one scallion on a flat surface, place $\frac{1}{4}$ of the beans across, pull up the scallion end, tie in a knot, and trim. Repeat the process with the remaining scallions and beans. Serve hot.

NOTES: These bundles make an excellent presentation on a dinner plate. You may substitute long strands of chives, softened for a few seconds in the microwave, for the scallions.

---

39 Calories; 1g Fat (24% CFF); 2g Protein; 6g Carbohydrate; 0mg Cholesterol; 39mg Sodium

Oven Roasted Potatoes

Serves: 4   Preparation Time: 1:00

Amount	Measure	Ingredient — Preparation Method
4	medium	russet potatoes — scrubbed
1	tablespoon	olive oil
1	tablespoon	salt free seasoning

Preheat oven to 400°. Lightly coat a jelly roll pan with vegetable cooking spray.

Cut the potatoes into bite-sized cubes. In a large bowl combine all ingredients tossing well to distribute the flavorings evenly. Place the potatoes on the pan in a single layer, spread so they do not touch each other.

Bake for 30 minutes, turn with a spatula and return to the oven for 15-20 minutes more or until crispy on the outside and tender inside. Serve hot.

313 Calories; 4g Fat (10% CFF); 7g Protein; 66g Carbohydrate; 0mg Cholesterol; 21mg Sodium

Skinny Mashed Potatoes

Serves: 4   Preparation Time: 0:25

Amount	Measure	Ingredient — Preparation Method
2 ½	pounds	potatoes — peeled, cubed
¼	cup	low sodium chicken broth — warmed
½	cup	fat free half and half — warmed
		salt & pepper — to taste

Bring 4 cups of water and potatoes to a boil in a 2-quart saucepan. Boil gently for 15-20 minutes or until tender. Drain and mash. Add the remaining ingredients gradually to obtain the desired consistency and taste. Serve hot.

NOTES: This recipe came from the label of a can of low sodium chicken broth. They are right in suggesting that a small amount of broth gives mashed potatoes a buttery sheen without the butter fat.

Try the yellow-gold variety of potatoes for a rich, buttery look.

190 Calories; 1g Fat (1% CFF); 6g Protein; 42g Carbohydrate; 0mg Cholesterol; 61mg Sodium

Roasted Honey-Mustard Potatoes

Serves: 4   Preparation Time: 0:55

Amount	Measure	Ingredient — Preparation Method
2	tablespoons	grainy Dijon mustard
1	tablespoon	honey
$\frac{1}{8}$	teaspoon	black pepper
1	tablespoon	canola oil
2	cups	russet potatoes — scrubbed, cubed
2	cups	sweet potatoes — peeled, cubed

Preheat oven to 400°. Lightly coat a jelly roll pan with vegetable cooking spray.

In a large bowl combine the mustard, honey, pepper and oil. Stir in the potato cubes and coat evenly. Spread the mixture in a single layer on the prepared jelly roll pan.

Roast for 25 minutes, turn with a spatula and roast an additional 15-20 minutes or until fork-tender on the inside and crispy on the outside.

NOTES: The old-fashioned whole seed mustard gives this dish great texture and eye appeal as do the two colors of potatoes.

217 Calories; 4g Fat (16% CFF); 4g Protein; 44g Carbohydrate; 0mg Cholesterol; 166mg Sodium

Brian's Potato Latkes

Serves: 4   Preparation Time: 0:30

Amount	Measure	Ingredient — Preparation Method
3	medium	potatoes — peeled
1/4	cup	onions — peeled
1	cup	flour
1		egg
1/2	cup	non fat milk
1/8	teaspoon	salt

Using a box grater or the fine grating blade of a food processor, grate the potatoes and onion. Add the remaining ingredients, stir until lump free.

Lightly coat a large griddle with vegetable cooking spray. Warm over medium heat until a drop of water dances across the surface.

Drop the batter by spoonfuls onto the griddle. After 3-4 minutes, when the latke tops begin to dry out and the bottoms are golden brown, turn and cook for another 2-3 minutes or until golden brown. Remove to a serving platter and keep warm. Repeat the process with the remaining batter. Delicious served with applesauce or maple syrup.

NOTES: If using a box grater, save your knuckles by securing a fork in the top one inch of the potato and hold firmly by the handle when grating. Use caution just in case it slips. Another method is to grip the potato with a (clean) rubber jar opener and grate carefully.

359 Calories; 2g Fat (5% CFF); 12g Protein; 75g Carbohydrate; 54mg Cholesterol; 115mg Sodium

Beautiful Potato Patties

Serves: 4   Preparation Time: 0:55

Amount	Measure	Ingredient — Preparation Method
4	medium	potatoes — peeled, cubed
1	cup	low sodium chicken broth — divided
1	cup	onions — chopped
$\frac{1}{4}$	medium	sweet red pepper — cut in thin strips
$\frac{1}{4}$	medium	green bell pepper — cut in thin strips
1		egg white — lightly beaten
1	teaspoon	olive oil

Bring 4 cups of water and the potatoes to a boil in a 3-quart saucepan. Boil gently for 8-10 minutes until tender. Drain, mash with half of the broth, then set aside to cool slightly. Meanwhile, pour some of the broth into a skillet and place over medium-high heat. Cook the onions in the broth until they soften and brown, about 15 minutes, adding more broth as needed. Just before they are done, push the onions off to the side of the skillet and then add the pepper strips to soften them in the remaining broth for about 1 minute. Remove from the heat, set aside.

Mix the egg white with the mashed potatoes and form into 4 oval patties about $\frac{1}{2}$" thick. Heat the oil in the skillet over medium heat, place the patties in the pan and press the pepper strips and onions into a decorative pattern on top. Cover and cook for 15 minutes or until the insides are piping hot and the bottoms are crispy brown.

NOTES: Save time by using leftover mashed potatoes. If the potatoes are cold from the refrigerator, then microwave them for 1-2 minutes before forming into patties.

318 Calories; 2g Fat (5% CFF); 9g Protein; 69g Carbohydrate; 0mg Cholesterol; 123mg Sodium

Potato Cheese Casserole

Serves: 4   Preparation Time: 1:05

Amount	Measure	Ingredient — Preparation Method
10	ounces	fat free cream of chicken soup, condensed
1	tablespoon	butter — grated
1	cup	reduced fat cheddar cheese — shredded
¼	cup	onions — chopped
½	cup	fat free sour cream
⅛	teaspoon	pepper
4	cups	shoestring hash browns, frozen — thawed
2	tablespoons	seasoned breadcrumbs
¼	teaspoon	paprika

Preheat oven to 375°. Lightly coat an 8" or 9" baking dish with vegetable cooking spray.

In a large bowl stir to blend the condensed soup, butter, cheese, onion, sour cream and pepper. Drain and fold in the potatoes. Spread the mixture evenly in the dish. Sprinkle with breadcrumbs and paprika.

Cover, bake for 30 minutes, uncover and bake for 25 minutes more or until golden brown.

NOTES: My mother-in-law may not recognize her original recipe here. By choosing the fat free versions of hash browned potatoes, cream of chicken soup and sour cream and the reduced fat version of cheddar cheese, the fat content of this recipe is one-quarter of the original. A mere shadow of its former self.

253 Calories; 11g Fat (39% CFF); 11g Protein; 27g Carbohydrate; 37mg Cholesterol; 921mg Sodium

Summer Potatoes

Serves: 4   Preparation Time: 0:55

Amount	Measure	Ingredient — Preparation Method
1	teaspoon	garlic — minced
$\frac{1}{2}$	teaspoon	salt free seasoning
$\frac{1}{8}$	teaspoon	salt substitute
1	tablespoon	brown sugar
2	tablespoons	fresh basil
2	teaspoons	olive oil
$\frac{1}{2}$	cup	onions — chopped
2	cups	red potatoes — scrubbed, cubed
1	cup	cherry tomatoes — cut in half

Preheat oven to 400°. Lightly coat a jelly roll pan with vegetable cooking spray.

In a large bowl combine all ingredients. Spread the mixture evenly in a single layer on the pan.

Roast for 45 minutes, turning occasionally with a spatula for even cooking. It is done when the potatoes are tender inside and slightly crispy outside.

NOTES: If fresh basil isn't available, substitute 1 teaspoon of dried basil.

79 Calories; 2g Fat (26% CFF); 1g Protein; 14g Carbohydrate; 0mg Cholesterol; 8mg Sodium

Potato Petals

Serves: 2   Preparation Time: 1:10

Amount	Measure	Ingredient — Preparation Method
1	large	russet potato — scrubbed
3/4	teaspoon	olive oil — divided
1/2	teaspoon	onion powder
1/8	teaspoon	black pepper
3	tablespoons	light sour cream
1/2	teaspoon	garlic — minced
2	teaspoons	grainy Dijon mustard
1	teaspoon	horseradish — prepared
2	tablespoons	reduced fat cheddar cheese — shredded
1	tablespoon	capers — rinsed, drained

Preheat oven to 400°. Using an 11" x 7" baking pan, brush half of the oil where the potatoes will lay, set aside.

Slice the potatoes into 30 thin rounds. Separate into 2 portions. Lay the slices in 2 tight circles on the pan to form flowers. Brush the remaining oil on the outer edges of the slices and sprinkle with onion powder and pepper. In a separate bowl combine the remaining ingredients. Spoon equal amounts of the mixture into the center of each "flower".

Cover, bake for about 50 minutes or until fork tender and brown and crispy underneath. Remove with a wide spatula.

NOTES: My favorite basting brush is the type with a slip collar that allows the bristles to spread easily for thorough cleaning. Any pastry brush sent through the dishwasher should be rinsed again under cold water to remove any dishwasher detergent that may have adhered to the bristles.

193 Calories; 4g Fat (18% CFF); 6g Protein; 35g Carbohydrate; 7mg Cholesterol; 215mg Sodium

Orange - Raisin Rice

Serves: 4   Preparation Time: 0:25

Amount	Measure	Ingredient — Preparation Method
2 ¼	cups	cold water
11	ounces	mandarin oranges — drained, use juice
¼	cup	raisins
1	cup	white rice
¼	cup	scallions — sliced thin

Bring the water, orange segments and raisins to a boil in a 2-quart saucepan. Add the rice, cover, reduce heat to low and simmer for 18-20 minutes or until all the liquid is absorbed. Fold in the scallions. Serve hot.

NOTES: To enhance the flavor use the drained liquid from the oranges as part of the water measurement.

Try Jasmine rice for a refreshing new taste.

223 Calories; 1g Fat (2% CFF); 4g Protein; 51g Carbohydrate; 0mg Cholesterol; 9mg Sodium

Lauren's Rice Pilaf

Serves: 4   Preparation Time: 0:30

Amount	Measure	Ingredient — Preparation Method
2	cups	low sodium chicken broth
1	cup	long-grain white rice
1/4	cup	sweet red peppers — chopped
1/4	cup	carrots — chopped
1/4	cup	onions — chopped
1	tablespoon	fresh parsley — chopped
1	teaspoon	salt free seasoning

Bring the broth to a boil in a 1-quart saucepan. Add the remaining ingredients. Cover, return to a boil then immediately reduce the heat to low, simmer for 20 minutes or until the liquid is absorbed. Fluff with a fork.

NOTES: Children and adults enjoy this rice pilaf and ask for it often. Add your family's favorite vegetables and watch them clean their plates!

203 Calories; 1g Fat (2% CFF); 9g Protein; 40g Carbohydrate; 0mg Cholesterol; 265mg Sodium

Lemon Barley Pilaf

Serves: 4   Preparation Time: 1:00

Amount	Measure	Ingredient — Preparation Method
3	cups	low sodium chicken broth
³⁄₄	cup	pearled barley
¹⁄₄	teaspoon	lemon peel — grated
¹⁄₄	whole	lemon — peeled, minced
¹⁄₄	cup	seedless raisins — chopped
¹⁄₄	cup	carrots — chopped
¹⁄₄	cup	onions — chopped

Bring the broth to a boil in a 2-quart saucepan. Add the remaining ingredients, cover, and reduce the heat to simmer, cook for 45 minutes. Remove from heat, let stand for 5 minutes.

NOTES: Pearled barley is a healthy alternative to rice or pasta. Similar to rice, it has had the bran removed and has been steamed and polished. We used the medium size for this recipe, although it is also available in coarse, fine and a quick-cooking type.

When using the peels of citrus fruit be sure to wash, rinse and dry the fruit before grating or peeling.

205 Calories; 1g Fat (2% CFF); 13g Protein; 40g Carbohydrate; 0mg Cholesterol; 396mg Sodium

Howie's Kasha Varnishkas

Serves: 4   Preparation Time: 0:25

Amount	Measure	Ingredient — Preparation Method
1	cup	pasta bowties
4	teaspoons	canola oil — divided
1	cup	onions — chopped
1	cup	buckwheat groats — medium grind
1		egg
½	teaspoon	salt
½	teaspoon	garlic powder
3	cups	boiling water

Cook pasta bowties according to package directions, drain. Meanwhile, using a heavy skillet warm 2 teaspoons of the oil over medium heat, add the onion and stir until golden brown, about 10 minutes. Remove the onions, add the remaining oil to the pan, add the buckwheat groats, stir for about 30 seconds or until the grain releases its fragrance and begins to pop. Meanwhile, in a small bowl beat the egg and seasonings, stir into the buckwheat groats. Using a spatula break up the pieces, cooking until dry and lump free. Add the boiling water, stir, cover tightly, reduce heat, and simmer for 12-15 minutes, until the liquid is absorbed. Fold in the cooked pasta and browned onions. Serve hot.

NOTES: I have Howie's caring wife to thank for the trimmed down version of this recipe.

Buckwheat groats, otherwise known as "kasha" are hulled, triangular seeds, sold either crushed or whole and cooked in the same way as rice. They are sold in fine, medium and coarse grinds and are available in the ethnic food aisle of most grocery stores.

314 Calories; 7g Fat (21% CFF); 10g Protein; 54g Carbohydrate; 53mg Cholesterol; 295mg Sodium

Lemon Pasta

Serves: 4   Preparation Time: 0:30

Amount	Measure	Ingredient — Preparation Method
8	ounces	pasta
1	pound	asparagus — trimmed
1	tablespoon	olive oil
$\frac{1}{4}$	teaspoon	garlic powder
$\frac{1}{8}$	teaspoon	black pepper
2	teaspoons	lemon peel — grated
3	tablespoons	lemon juice
1	cup	black beans, cooked — rinsed, drained
2	tablespoons	pine nuts (pignoli) — lightly toasted
4	tablespoons	parmesan cheese — grated

Boil the pasta in a 2-quart saucepan until almost done. Cut the asparagus into bite-sized pieces. 2 minutes before the pasta is done, add the asparagus, cover and boil gently for 1 minute, drain. Meanwhile, in a large bowl combine the olive oil, garlic powder, pepper, lemon peel and juice. Fold in the pasta, asparagus and the remaining ingredients. Serve hot.

NOTES: Toast the pine nuts in a toaster oven for 1 minute until fragrant and lightly browned for this delicately flavored dish.

364 Calories; 9g Fat (21% CFF); 16g Protein; 57g Carbohydrate; 4mg Cholesterol; 99mg Sodium

DESSERTS AND BREADS

Cheryl Mochau

Chocolate Butterscotch Cookies

Serves: 26   Preparation Time: 0:35

Amount	Measure	Ingredient — Preparation Method
1	cup	sugar
$\frac{1}{2}$	cup	cocoa powder
$\frac{3}{4}$	cup	flour
$\frac{1}{2}$	teaspoon	baking soda
$\frac{1}{2}$	cup	butterscotch chips
2		egg whites
$\frac{1}{4}$	cup	applesauce
1	teaspoon	vanilla extract

Preheat oven to 375°. Line 2 cookie sheets with parchment paper, set aside.

In a large bowl combine the sugar, cocoa, flour, baking soda and butterscotch chips. In another bowl beat the egg whites briskly with a wire whisk until foamy, about 30 seconds. Beat in the applesauce and vanilla. Pour the wet ingredients into the dry ingredients, stirring just enough to blend. Drop by tablespoonfuls onto the prepared cookie sheets.

Bake for 10-12 minutes or until puffy and slightly dry around the edges. Cool on a wire rack.

NOTES: Parchment paper makes baking almost foolproof. The reusable heavy paper creates a buffer from metal pans that would otherwise scorch and cause the food to stick. It's available in major grocery stores and kitchen shops. Other uses are for baking en papillote (in paper) and, when folded correctly, for use as disposable pastry bags.

63 Calories; 1g Fat (5% CFF); 1g Protein; 15g Carbohydrate; 0mg Cholesterol; 30mg Sodium

Anne's Butterscotch Meringues

Serves: 24 Preparation Time: 0:45

Amount	Measure	Ingredient — Preparation Method
4		egg whites
1/4	teaspoon	salt
1/4	teaspoon	cream of tartar
3/4	teaspoon	vanilla powder
3/4	cup	granulated sugar
8	ounces	butterscotch chips

Preheat oven to 300°. Line 2 cookie sheets with parchment paper, set aside.

Beat the egg whites, salt, cream of tartar and vanilla powder until soft peaks begin to form. Add the sugar gradually, beating until stiff. Fold in the butterscotch chips. Drop by teaspoonfuls onto the prepared pans.

Bake for about 25 minutes or until dry. To store, wait until completely cool and then stack between layers of waxed paper and cover tightly. Makes 48.

NOTES: This recipe came from The Boston Globe's Chatter's column.

Don't try to make meringues on a humid day unless you are in an air-conditioned kitchen, otherwise they won't dry properly and will feel tacky.

65 Calories; 1g Fat (5% CFF); 1g Protein; 15g Carbohydrate; 1mg Cholesterol; 35mg Sodium

Baked Apples Shafer

Serves: 8   Preparation Time: 0:50

Amount	Measure	Ingredient — Preparation Method
2	large	Granny Smith apples
2	large	Rome apples
$\frac{1}{3}$	cup	brown sugar
$\frac{1}{3}$	cup	raisins
1	tablespoon	flour
1	teaspoon	cinnamon
$\frac{1}{2}$	teaspoon	vanilla powder

Preheat oven to 400°.

Scrub then cut the apples in half from top to bottom, remove the core, sharp stems and blossom ends. In a separate bowl combine the remaining ingredients. Spoon the mixture into each apple cavity.

Place the apples in a 9" x 13" x 2" baking pan, add 2 cups of hot water, cover tightly, then bake for 40 minutes or until tender when pierced with a toothpick.

NOTES: Use a melon baller to remove the core and a paring knife to trim rough stem ends.

To prevent the apples from bursting open during baking, cut a few small nicks in the skin before baking.

Vanilla powder is available wherever most cake decorating supplies are sold.

94 Calories; 1g Fat (2% CFF); 0.5g Protein; 24g Carbohydrate; 0mg Cholesterol; 5mg Sodium

Cherry Bread Pudding

Serves: 9   Preparation Time: 1:10

Amount	Measure	Ingredient — Preparation Method
1	cup	egg substitute
1	cup	sugar
1	tablespoon	vanilla extract
2	cups	non fat milk
5	cups	bread — cut into pieces
1	cup	cherry pie filling

Preheat oven to 375°. Lightly coat a 2-quart baking dish with vegetable cooking spray.

Using a wire whisk, blend the egg substitute and sugar until the sugar dissolves. Add the vanilla and milk, continue whisking for 30 seconds. Submerge the bread cubes in the liquid and pour into the prepared baking dish. Drop 9 spoonfuls of cherry pie filling over the top, pushing it partially down into the bread mixture.

Bake for 1 hour or until golden brown and firm when gently shaken.

NOTES: This recipe uses up every scrap of bread from the Shrimp Toast recipe found elsewhere in this book.

Egg substitutes make this dessert a healthier treat for those who need to reduce cholesterol, but still want comfort food. If desired, substitute 8 large egg whites for one cup of egg substitute.

535 Calories; 8g Fat (13% CFF); 16g Protein; 99g Carbohydrate; 3mg Cholesterol; 791mg Sodium

Extra Energy Hermit Bars

Serves: 16   Preparation Time: 0:30

Amount	Measure	Ingredient — Preparation Method
½	cup	granulated sugar
1 ½	cups	flour
½	teaspoon	baking powder
1	teaspoon	baking soda
2	tablespoons	pumpkin pie spice
½	cup	apples — minced
¼	cup	raisins — chopped
¼	cup	molasses
1		egg
2	tablespoons	cider vinegar

Preheat oven to 350°. Lightly coat an 11" x 15" jelly roll pan with vegetable cooking spray.

In a large bowl combine the sugar, flour, baking powder, baking soda and spice. Stir in the fruit and coat completely. In a separate bowl combine the molasses, egg and vinegar. Add it to the flour mixture and blend thoroughly. Spread the batter in long rows, ¼" thick by 2" wide. Leave 2" between the rows. Bake for 15 minutes. Cool on wire racks. Cut into bars.

NOTES: Sprinkle a little sugar on top of these before baking for a crispier top.

97 Calories; 1g Fat (5% CFF); 2g Protein; 22g Carbohydrate; 13mg Cholesterol; 97mg Sodium

Mary Ellen's 4th of July Trifle

Serves: 12   Preparation Time: 0:15

Amount	Measure	Ingredient — Preparation Method
3	ounces	vanilla instant pudding mix
1	cup	light sour cream
1	cup	2% low fat milk
1	tablespoon	grated orange peel
2	cups	non dairy whipped topping, light — thawed
12	ounces	ladyfinger cookies
2	pints	fresh strawberries — trimmed, sliced
1	pint	fresh blueberries — picked clean

Combine the first 4 ingredients and beat at low speed with a mixer. Fold in the whipped topping, set aside. Using a trifle bowl or other large clear bowl, stand the ladyfingers around the circumference of the bowl, saving a few to break up for use as the second layer. Pour half of the pudding mixture into the bowl, straighten any leaning ladies and scatter the remaining broken cookies over the pudding. Saving several berries for garnish, sprinkle the berries evenly, then spread the remainder of the pudding on top. Level off with a spatula and garnish with the reserved berries.

NOTES: To make this extra rich and more authentic, my Aunt Mary Ellen sometimes beats real whipping cream with sugar and vanilla, instead of using the lower fat whipped topping. For an even more patriotic presentation, she often makes an American flag decoration on top with the remaining berries!

200 Calories; 5g Fat (22% CFF); 5g Protein; 34g Carbohydrate; 106mg Cholesterol; 173mg Sodium

Chocolate Strawberry Oat Bars

Serves: 16   Preparation Time: 1:00

Amount	Measure	Ingredient — Preparation Method
1	cup	flour
1	cup	rolled oats
2/3	cup	brown sugar — packed
1/2	cup	chocolate chips
1/2	teaspoon	baking powder
1/2	cup	non fat milk
2		egg whites
1/2	cup	applesauce
1	teaspoon	vanilla extract
1/2	cup	fresh strawberries — rinsed, sliced
1/4	cup	almonds — sliced
1/2	cup	confectioner's sugar
1/8	teaspoon	vanilla extract
3	tablespoons	non fat milk

Preheat oven to 350°. Lightly coat an 8" x 8" pan with vegetable cooking spray.

In a large bowl combine the flour, oats, brown sugar, chocolate chips and baking powder. In a separate bowl beat the milk, egg whites, applesauce and vanilla until frothy. Pour the wet ingredients into the dry ingredients, stir to blend. Spread the batter evenly in the pan, sprinkle with berries and almonds.
Bake for 45 minutes or until a cake tester inserted into the center comes out clean.

Icing: Combine the confectioner's sugar, vanilla and milk until the mixture drizzles in thin lines off the end of a spoon (adding more milk if needed). After the cake is cool, drizzle with icing and cut into bars.

NOTES: For best results, rinse and let the berries dry before slicing.

158 Calories; 4g Fat (20% CFF); 3g Protein; 29g Carbohydrate; 0mg Cholesterol; 29mg Sodium

Wheat Free Coffee Cake

Serves: 9   Preparation Time: 1:10

Amount	Measure	Ingredient — Preparation Method
²⁄₃	cup	non fat milk
1	tablespoon	lemon juice
1	cup	white rice flour
¹⁄₃	cup	potato starch flour
1	teaspoon	xanthan gum
¹⁄₂	teaspoon	baking powder
¹⁄₂	teaspoon	baking soda
¹⁄₈	teaspoon	salt
2		eggs
³⁄₄	cup	sugar
¹⁄₄	cup	applesauce
1	teaspoon	vanilla extract
¹⁄₄	cup	brown sugar
1	teaspoon	cinnamon
1	tablespoon	butter — cut in small bits
2	tablespoons	white rice flour
¹⁄₄	cup	walnuts — chopped
1	cup	confectioner's sugar
2	tablespoons	non fat milk
¹⁄₈	teaspoon	vanilla extract

Preheat oven to 350°. Lightly coat an 8" x 8" cake pan with vegetable cooking spray, dust with rice flour and set aside.

Combine the milk and lemon juice, stir and set aside. Sift together the rice flour, potato starch, xanthan gum, baking powder, baking soda and salt, set aside. Using a large bowl and mixer, beat the eggs on medium-high for 30 seconds, add the sugar, applesauce and vanilla and continue beating for 45 seconds or until the mixture is light in color and slightly thickened. Slowly alternate between adding the dry ingredients and the reserved "buttermilk" to the egg mixture. Beat at medium speed until the batter is free of lumps and pale yellow in color. Spoon into the prepared cake pan.

Topping: In a separate bowl combine the brown sugar, cinnamon, butter, rice flour and walnuts. Sprinkle evenly on top of the cake. Bake for 50 minutes or until a toothpick inserted in the center comes out clean.

Icing: Meanwhile, prepare a thin icing by blending the confectioner's sugar, milk and vanilla. When the cake is done, remove from the oven, cool and drizzle the icing over the top. Cut into squares.

NOTES: The non fat milk and lemon juice create a "buttermilk" substitute, which acts as a thickening agent, while applesauce replaces the oil in the batter.

When using cold or frozen butter, grate it to make blending easier.

Xanthan gum, a.k.a. xantham gum, acts as a gluten substitute in wheat free baking. Without it, breads and cakes would lack elasticity and crumble.

300 Calories; 5g Fat (14% CFF); 5g Protein; 61g Carbohydrate; 52mg Cholesterol; 163mg Sodium

Vanilla Cheesecake

Serves: 10   Preparation Time: 1:45

Amount	Measure	Ingredient — Preparation Method
1	cup	graham cracker crumbs
		spray margarine — shake well
2	whole	eggs
3		egg whites
1	cup	sugar
16	ounces	fat free cream cheese — cut in cubes
8	ounces	low fat cottage cheese
8	ounces	low fat vanilla yogurt
3	tablespoons	cornstarch
3	tablespoons	flour
1	tablespoon	lemon juice
1 ½	tablespoons	vanilla extract

Preheat oven to 400°F. Lightly coat a 9" springform pan with vegetable cooking spray.

Place crumbs in the pan, level off and spray with margarine (about 10 pump sprays). Press down firmly to form a compact crust. Bake for 5 minutes then remove to cool.

In a food processor fitted with a chopping blade (or with an electric mixer), beat the eggs until pale yellow and light, while gradually adding sugar. Continue mixing, adding cream cheese in small bits until smooth. Add the remaining ingredients one at a time. Stop to scrape the sides and bottom of the bowl occasionally, then continue beating until the mixture is free of lumps. Pour into the cake pan.

Place the pan in a hot water bath and bake for 15 minutes at 400°F. Without opening the oven door, reduce the oven temperature to 300° and bake for one hour. The cake may be slightly loose in the center, but it should firm up as it cools. To prevent cracking, do not remove the cake from the hot water bath until after it has cooled considerably. If possible, leave the cake in the oven with the door ajar as it cools.

NOTES: To prevent the hot water bath from seeping into the cake, I usually place the springform pan into another slightly larger pan before setting it in the water. All it takes is a slight bend in the pan to create a leak, and then you're stuck with a soggy cake. Lest you consider eliminating the hot water bath altogether, remember that its function is to create moisture so the cake doesn't end up dry with gaping cracks in the top.

241 Calories; 2g Fat (9% CFF); 13g Protein; 38g Carbohydrate; 52mg Cholesterol; 427mg Sodium

Lemon Tarts

Serves: 12   Preparation Time: 0:45

Amount	Measure	Ingredient — Preparation Method
1		egg
3/4	cup	sugar
2	tablespoons	cornstarch
1/3	cup	water
1/3	cup	lemon juice
2	cups	corn flakes
1	cup	coconut flakes
1/2	cup	sugar
1/4	cup	flour
1	teaspoon	vanilla extract
2		egg whites
1/2	cup	non dairy whipped topping, light

Filling: Lightly beat the egg in a bowl, set aside. Combine the sugar and cornstarch in a 2-quart saucepan. Add water and lemon juice, whisk to dissolve. Bring to a boil, reduce heat to medium, and beat for 30 seconds. Using a wire whisk, beat the egg in the bowl briskly while pouring the hot lemon mixture in a very thin stream into it. Return the lemon and egg mixture to the heat, cook for 1 minute, stirring constantly. Remove from the heat, set aside to cool.

Crust: Preheat oven to 350°. Coat 24 mini muffin cups with vegetable cooking spray.

Lightly crush the corn flakes to equal 1 cup and combine with the coconut, sugar, flour, vanilla and egg whites. Divide the dough equally in the muffin cups, then press into the bottom and up the sides of each cup. Bake for 20 minutes or until crusty, brown and fragrant. If the centers have risen while baking and lost most of their indent, press them down with the back of spoon while still hot. Remove to cool on wire racks.

When completely cool, fill each shell with the lemon filling and a dollop of non dairy whipped topping. Refrigerate until serving. Makes 24 mini tarts.

NOTES: For best results make these at least 3 hours prior to serving to allow time for the shells and filling to chill completely.

158 Calories; 3g Fat (16% CFF); 2g Protein; 32g Carbohydrate; 18mg Cholesterol; 80mg Sodium

Pumpkin Noodle Kugel

Serves: 4   Preparation Time: 0:50

Amount	Measure	Ingredient — Preparation Method
½	cup	egg substitute
1	cup	non fat milk
½	cup	sugar
2	teaspoons	vanilla extract
½	teaspoon	pumpkin pie spice
8	ounces	pumpkin, canned
¼	cup	raisins
3	ounces	egg noodles, fat free

Preheat oven to 400°. Lightly coat a 1-½-quart baking dish with vegetable cooking spray.

In a large bowl combine everything except the egg noodles. Stir thoroughly to dissolve the sugar. Fold in the uncooked egg noodles. Pour the mixture into the baking dish.

Cover and bake at 400° for 30 minutes. Remove the cover and bake an additional 10-15 minutes or until light brown and the center moves only slightly when gently shaken.

NOTES: The uncooked egg noodles will soften and cook as they absorb the liquids in this recipe.

4 large egg whites equals ½ cup of egg substitute.

299 Calories; 4g Fat (12% CFF); 9g Protein; 57g Carbohydrate; 2mg Cholesterol; 107mg Sodium

Anadama Bread

Serves: 12   Preparation Time: 2:25

Amount	Measure	Ingredient — Preparation Method
3 ¼	cups	flour — divided
¼	cup	cornmeal
1	package	dry yeast, fast acting
¼	cup	dark molasses
1	cup	water
1	teaspoon	salt
2	tablespoons	canola oil
1	whole	egg

Using the large bowl of an electric mixer, combine 1 ½ cups flour, the cornmeal and yeast, set aside. In a 1-quart saucepan warm the molasses, water, salt and oil to tepid (115°-120°). Add the liquid to the dry ingredients, add the egg, and beat by hand to combine. Gradually add 1 ½ cups of flour and stir to combine. Knead for 3 minutes by hand, or use the dough hook and low setting on an electric mixer. Add ¼ cup (more or less) of flour while kneading to prevent sticking.

Cover the bowl with plastic wrap, set in a warm place to rise until double in bulk. Meanwhile, lightly coat a 9" x 5" x 3" loaf pan with vegetable cooking spray, set aside. Punch down the dough then place in the prepared pan. Cover, let rise until almost to the top of the pan.

Bake in a 375° oven for 35-40 minutes or until it smells incredible and makes a hollow sound when tapped.

NOTES: Get the molasses moving faster by warming the open jar in the microwave oven for 10-20 seconds before measuring.

Sulphured or unsulphured molasses? Sulphur is sometimes used in molasses processing, where it imparts a slightly 'heavier' taste than the unsulphered molasses.

181 Calories; 3g Fat (16% CFF); 5g Protein; 33g Carbohydrate; 18mg Cholesterol; 191mg Sodium

Elegant Pear Sauté

Serves: 4   Preparation Time: 0:20

Amount	Measure	Ingredient — Preparation Method
1	cup	fresh squeezed orange juice
4	small	Bosc pears
1	teaspoon	butter
3	tablespoons	sugar
1	tablespoon	cornstarch
3	tablespoons	cold water
2	teaspoons	vanilla extract
¼	teaspoon	almond extract
4	sprigs	mint
1	tablespoon	grated orange peel

Pour the orange juice into a medium bowl. Peel and slice the pears thin, dropping them into the juice to coat. Drain the juice off into a large skillet, add the butter and sugar, and bring to a boil. Add the pears, reduce the heat to simmer for about 5 minutes. Turn the pears over to cook evenly for another 4 minutes or just until tender. In a small cup combine the cornstarch with the cold water. Blend into the simmering liquid. Stir to thicken slightly. Remove from the heat, add the vanilla and almond extracts. Stir to blend the flavors. Serve with a garnish of mint sprigs and grated orange peel.

NOTES: This is the same recipe that was printed in the October 1998 Yankee magazine article about my personal cheffing business in Massachusetts: "Isn't There Somebody Who Could Come In and Cook?" written by Barbara Pierce.

173 Calories; 2g Fat (8% CFF); 1g Protein; 40g Carbohydrate; 3mg Cholesterol; 11mg Sodium

Easy Apple Crisp

Serves: 8   Preparation Time: 1:00

Amount	Measure	Ingredient — Preparation Method
4	cups	apples — peeled, sliced
2	teaspoons	pumpkin pie spice
1	teaspoon	sugar
³⁄₄	cup	applesauce
1	cup	reduced fat buttermilk baking mix
³⁄₄	cup	sugar
1		egg
¹⁄₂	cup	malted cereal granules
3	tablespoons	brown sugar

Preheat oven to 350°F.

Place apples in an ungreased 9" pie plate. Combine the pumpkin pie spice and 1 teaspoon of sugar, then sprinkle over the apples. In a medium bowl combine the applesauce, baking mix, sugar and egg. Spread evenly over the apples. Sprinkle with the cereal and brown sugar.

Bake for 45 minutes or until a cake tester inserted into the center comes out clean.

NOTES: If you're watching your cholesterol closely, then substitute two egg whites in place of the whole egg.

Malted cereal granules are the generic name for Grape-Nuts® cereal.

234 Calories; 2g Fat (8% CFF); 3g Protein; 54g Carbohydrate; 26mg Cholesterol; 250mg Sodium

Chocolate Tofu Pudding

Serves: 4   Preparation Time: 0:05

Amount	Measure	Ingredient — Preparation Method
16	ounces	soft silken tofu
¾	cup	sugar
½	cup	unsweetened cocoa powder
1	teaspoon	vanilla extract
¼	teaspoon	almond extract

Put the tofu and sugar in a food processor bowl fitted with a chopping blade. Blend for 20 seconds, stop, scrape the sides and blend for another 30 seconds to dissolve the sugar. Add the remaining ingredients. Blend for 20 seconds. Serve chilled.

NOTES: Silken tofu has a smooth custard-like texture and is best used to make puddings, pies and smoothies. It needn't be cooked to taste great, so long as strong flavors are added to compensate for its blandness.

260 Calories; 3g Fat (11% CFF); 6g Protein; 58g Carbohydrate; 0mg Cholesterol; 12mg Sodium

Honey Oat Muffins

Serves: 12 Preparation Time: 0:30

Amount	Measure	Ingredient — Preparation Method
1	cup	flour
2	teaspoons	baking powder
½	teaspoon	salt
1	cup	oatmeal
2		egg whites
1	cup	non fat milk
⅓	cup	applesauce
¼	cup	honey
½	teaspoon	vanilla extract
¼	cup	strawberry jam

Preheat oven to 400°. Lightly coat 12 muffin cups with vegetable cooking spray.

In a large bowl sift together the flour, baking powder and salt, then stir in the oatmeal and set aside. In a separate bowl blend the egg whites, milk, applesauce, honey and vanilla. Stir the wet ingredients into the dry ingredients. Blend just until moistened. Let stand for 3 minutes. Fill the muffin cups ⅓ full with batter, drop a teaspoon of jam in the center of each and the remaining batter on top.

Bake for 15-20 minutes until golden brown and the tops spring back when lightly pressed.

NOTES: For a little extra fiber and eye appeal, sprinkle the tops with oatmeal before baking.

118 Calories; 1g Fat (4% CFF); 4g Protein; 25g Carbohydrate; 0mg Cholesterol; 241mg Sodium

Treble Clef Breadsticks

Serves: 12   Preparation Time: 0:40

Amount	Measure	Ingredient — Preparation Method
8	ounces	bread dough, prepared
3	tablespoons	cornmeal
1	tablespoon	onion powder
1	tablespoon	caraway seed
1	tablespoon	parmesan cheese — shredded
2	tablespoons	milk
1	tablespoon	sesame seeds
1	tablespoon	kosher salt — optional

On a dry surface roll out the bread dough and cut into 12 equal portions (sprinkle a small amount of white flour if the dough is sticky). Roll each portion into a long rope and let rest for 5 minutes.

Scatter the cornmeal on a large cookie sheet, set aside.

In a small cup, combine the onion powder, caraway seeds and cheese. Sprinkle a small amount of the mixture on a dry surface and roll each dough rope out long and thin. Place each rope on the baking sheet by coiling it into the shape of a treble clef. Repeat the process until all of the seasonings and dough are used up. Baste milk on each one with a pastry brush then sprinkle sesame seeds and kosher salt (if desired) on top.

Move an oven rack to the middle of the oven. Preheat oven to 375°. Place the prepared bread sticks on top of the oven to rise slightly while it preheats.

Bake for 12-15 minutes or until golden brown.

NOTES: Choir members and musicians will feel honored and loved when they see these custom-made breadsticks. Choose from a wide variety of bread doughs available in chilled display cases at most grocery stores. Read the labels and make healthy choices!

79 Calories; 3g Fat (36% CFF); 2g Protein; 11g Carbohydrate; 1mg Cholesterol; 689mg Sodium

Barb's Wheat Free Bread

Serves: 16   Preparation Time: 2:30

Amount	Measure	Ingredient — Preparation Method
1 ½	cups	buttermilk
¼	cup	sugar
3	tablespoons	butter
1	teaspoon	salt
1	cup	white rice flour
1	cup	brown rice flour
¼	cup	tapioca flour
2 ¼	teaspoons	dry yeast, fast acting
2	teaspoons	xanthan gum
2		eggs

Using a 1-quart saucepan over medium heat, warm the buttermilk, sugar, butter and salt until the butter just begins to melt (120°-130°). Meanwhile, in a large mixing bowl sift together the flours, yeast and xanthan gum. Pour the liquid into the dry ingredients, add the eggs and whisk to blend. Cover and let rise in a warm place until doubled in bulk.

Lightly coat a 9" x 5" x 3" loaf pan with vegetable cooking spray. Stir the batter to reduce in size, pour into the loaf pan. Cover and let rise until the batter rises almost to the top of the loaf pan.

Preheat oven to 375°. Bake for 30-35 minutes if using a glass pan, or 40-45 minutes for a metal pan. The bread is done when it's golden brown and makes a hollow sound when tapped. Remove to cool on a wire rack and wait at least 30 minutes before slicing.

NOTES: There are 2 ¼ teaspoons in a ¼ ounce packet of dry yeast.

133 Calories; 3g Fat (23% CFF); 4g Protein; 22g Carbohydrate; 34mg Cholesterol; 189mg Sodium

Breakfast Pudding

Serves: 4   Preparation Time: 0:10

Amount	Measure	Ingredient — Preparation Method
1	cup	cooked rice
½	cup	cantaloupe — cubed
½	cup	strawberries — cut in half
½	cup	blueberries — rinsed, picked clean
1	cup	low fat vanilla yogurt
⅛	teaspoon	almond extract

Combine all ingredients in a large bowl, saving a few berries for garnish (if desired). Spoon into serving dishes. Serve chilled.

NOTES: Use leftover plain rice, barley or couscous with your favorite combination of fresh fruits and yogurt to personalize this recipe.

133 Calories; 1g Fat (7% CFF); 4g Protein; 27g Carbohydrate; 3mg Cholesterol; 41mg Sodium

Fruit & Honey Breakfast Bake

Serves: 8   Preparation Time: 0:50

Amount	Measure	Ingredient — Preparation Method
1 ½	cups	rolled oats
¼	cup	dried apricots — pitted, cut in half
¼	cup	dried plums — pitted, cut in half
¼	cup	sugar
2	teaspoons	vanilla extract
¼	teaspoon	almond extract
3	cups	non fat milk
½	cup	honey

Preheat oven to 375°. Lightly coat a 2-quart baking dish with vegetable cooking spray.

Combine the oats, dried apricots, dried plums and sugar in a large bowl. Add the vanilla extract, almond extract and milk, stir until lump-free. Pour the mixture into the baking dish, cover tightly and bake for 30 minutes.

Remove from the oven, uncover carefully, drizzle the honey on top, then bake uncovered for an additional 10 minutes.

NOTES: Delicious served hot or cold, with or without milk.

Dried plums — the fruit formerly known as prunes — have followed dairy products in changing their names to gain a new identity for the new millennium.

205 Calories; 1g Fat (5% CFF); 6g Protein; 44g Carbohydrate; 2mg Cholesterol; 49mg Sodium

Bibliography

Over the years many people have influenced me, including cookbook authors, celebrity chefs, food writers, clients, friends, and family. Those who have had the greatest impact as sources of information and inspiration are listed below — with apologies to any that have been omitted:

Martha Stewart, *Entertaining* (Clarkson N. Potter, 1982) — along with many of her other books.

Nathan Pritikin, *The Pritikin Program for Diet and Exercise* (Grosset & Dunlap, c. 1979).

Bobbie Hinman and Millie Snyder, the *Lean & Luscious* series of cookbooks (Prima Publishing, 1987).

Evelyn Tribole, M.S., R.D., *Healthy Homestyle Cooking* (Rodale Press, 1994).

Dean Ornish, M.D., *Everyday Cooking with Dr. Dean Ornish* (HarperCollins, 1996).

Julia Child, *The Way to Cook* (Alfred A. Knopf, 1989).

Lynn Fisher, *Healthy Indulgences* (Avon, 1997).

Carol Fenster, Ph.D., *Special Diet Solutions* (Savory Palate, 1997).

The Low-Fat Way To Cook (Oxmoor House, 1995).

Betty Crocker's 50th Anniversary Creative Recipes (General Mills, 1980).

Sharon Tyler Herbst, *Food Lover's Companion* (Barron's, 1990).

Cooking Light magazines.

Cook's Illustrated magazines.

Cooking friends from the Hospitality teams of AHCC, Tabernacle, and Christian Fellowship Churches.

My husband, Geoff, and the extended Mochau clan.

To all these people — and more — I extend my thanks!

Cheryl.

Cheryl Mochau

About The Author

Cheryl Young Mochau began her professional food career with a national hotel chain in 1985. Six years – and many covers – later she decided to strike out on her own as a personal chef in West Hartford, Connecticut.

"The 90's were a great time to cook for individuals and families. People seemed to really enjoy the latest food trends and to this day the low fat food revolution is still reflected in my cooking," says Cheryl.

The art of using lower fat cooking techniques predominates Cheryl's cooking for her personal chef clients, her cooking classes and even her consulting sessions with aspiring personal chefs.

In this her first book, *A Personal Chef Cooks: Recipes from a Decade of Lower Fat Cooking*, Cheryl shares the tastes and joys of one hundred recipes that have brought pleasure to dozens of client families over the years.

Cheryl now lives and operates her personal chef service, Cheryl Really Cooks! (online at: http://www.cherylreallycooks.com), in southwestern Indiana.

Printed in the United States
86134LV00013BB/58/A